T0110769

ALZHEIMER'S

Answers to Hard Questions for Families

By the same authors
The Patient in the Family

Alzheimer's

ANSWERS TO HARD QUESTIONS FOR FAMILIES

James Lindemann Nelson

AND

Hilde Lindemann Nelson

DOUBLEDAY

New York   London   Toronto   Sydney   Auckland

A MAIN STREET BOOK
PUBLISHED BY DOUBLEDAY
a division of Bantam Doubleday Dell Publishing Group, Inc.
1540 Broadway, New York, New York 10036

MAIN STREET BOOKS, DOUBLEDAY, and the portrayal of a building
with a tree are trademarks of Doubleday, a division of Bantam
Doubleday Dell Publishing Group, Inc.

Alzheimer's was originally published in hardcover by Doubleday
in 1996.
The Main Street Books edition is published by arrangement with
Doubleday.

The Library of Congress has cataloged the Doubleday edition
as follows:

Nelson, James Lindemann.
Alzheimer's: Answers to hard questions for families
James Lindemann Nelson and Hilde Lindemann Nelson.
p.   cm.
Includes bibliographical references.
1. Alzheimer's disease—Popular works. 2. Alzheimer's disease—
Patients—Family relationships. 3. Caregivers.
I. Nelson, Hilde Lindemann. II. Title.
RC523.2.N45   1996
382.1'96831—dc20   96-12567
CIP

ISBN 978-0-385-48534-0

146864218

Acknowledgments

WE WROTE THIS BOOK between 1993 and 1995, when we were both employed by the Hastings Center. For going on thirty years now, the center has been a leader in the important task of trying to understand better and meet responsibly the challenges society faces from changes in medical technology and health care practice. We are grateful to our former colleagues for many kinds of assistance, and pleased that our book can claim a place in the Hastings Center tradition.

While at Hastings, our research and writing were generously supported by a grant to the center from the Greenwall Foundation. Greenwall is one of the very few philanthropic organizations to make inquiry into the ethical implications of health care a major funding priority; we appreciate its wisdom in this general respect, as well as its particular interest in our project.

We have also had the help of two kinds of consultants. One was a group of professionals in the fields of aging, elder law, social work, philosophy, and nursing home administration. We'd like to thank Marjorie Cantor, an anthropologist from the Third Age Center of Fordham University; Bartholomew Collopy, a Fordham professor of humanities, also associated with the Third Age Center; Richard T. Hull, professor of philosophy at the State University of New York at Buffalo; Harry R. Moody, the deputy director of the Brookdale Center on Aging at Hunter College; Barbara Silverstone, a social worker and president of The Light House in New York City; Peter Strauss, a lawyer specializing in elder law; Connie Zuckerman, also a lawyer and coordinator of legal studies at the SUNY Health Science Center; and most especially thanks to Tony Yang-Lewis, director of the Alzheimer's Unit at Cobble Hill Nursing Home, Brooklyn, who found most of our family caregivers for us and was invaluable in coordinating our many meetings with them. Special thanks also to Carolyn Ells, a graduate student in philosophy at the University of Tennessee, whose help was invaluable in the final stages of preparing the manuscript.

The other, even more important group of consultants was, of course, the family caregivers who advised us, told us their stories, and read every chapter, sometimes several times, pointing out where we had missed an important point or where the writing wasn't readable enough. Their stories are not the ones told here, but we could not have told these stories well without their help. To Robin Benoff, Bessie Blow, Helen Broder, Doris Brunsen, Roberta Burke, Judith Carlin, Eleanor Glass, Helen Glassman, Judy Knipe, Robert Kushner, Sylvia Mosola, Rita and Darren Pearl, Evelyn and Frank Roselle, Willie Senders, Shirley Spain, Lenore and Neil Stoller, Susan Sugarman, Catherine Unsino, Aurora and John Walton, Sandy Weisman, Paula Westho, and Howard Wolk, our deepest thanks for all your help and apologies for anything we still didn't get right. We dedicate this book to you.

HILDE LINDEMANN NELSON
JAMES LINDEMANN NELSON
Knoxville, 1996

Contents

ALZHEIMER'S

Answers to
Hard Questions
for Families

Introduction

Moral Troubles

AN EXHAUSTED, middle-aged woman stands in the bedroom doorway as the gray light of early morning outlines her father, asleep under the quilt. Barbara Kessler Johnson is just about drained. As she pulls her robe more tightly about her, she feels that with this gesture she is also holding herself together. Her dad, diagnosed several years ago as having Alzheimer's disease, is starting to stir, and she is dreading the moment when he will awake. It's not the "how-to" problems that are getting her down—how to get him to the bathroom, how to improve his appetite—it's the moral problems.

Mr. Kessler begins every morning by sitting up in bed and asking for his wife, who has been dead these twelve years. Barbara has learned the hard way that if she tells him the truth, however gently, however matter-of-factly, her father's grief will be as deep as if the loss were fresh. To him it *is* fresh, every time. Yet, if she tells a lie—if she says that her mother is out shopping, or visiting, or at work—she may have to fend off his questions all day long, piling further lies on top of the first one. Her father is not so demented that he always accepts what he's told without question; if she lies, he's likely to be suspicious and sometimes flat-out nasty, blaming his daughter for keeping his wife from him.

Barbara is profoundly tired of wrestling with this problem, and with all the other problems he causes as well. The refrain that's been running through her head for months starts up again: Dad really should be in a nursing home. But shortly after he was finally diagnosed, he asked her repeatedly to promise that she would never "turn him out of his own house." She gave him her word, and meant it. Of course, when she made that promise, Barbara didn't know what she knows now. She didn't know how hard it would be to take care of him. She didn't know that she'd be facing life without her own husband, who left her two years before to marry a woman both younger and unburdened by a demented father. And while she didn't have great hopes of her brothers, she didn't know they would leave virtually all of Dad's care to her.

As Barbara and tens of thousands of other family caregivers have discovered, a diagnosis of Alzheimer's or another dementing disease is devastating news, not only for the person suffering from it but for everyone who is "in close": spouse, children, nieces, nephews, and sometimes parents. People with these illnesses and their families feel despair and helplessness in the face of a future that seems full of terrible and altogether unavoidable problems.

Some of these problems are, of course, medical ones. Many dementias—Alzheimer's in particular—are difficult to *diagnose*. Family physicians too often pass off the symptoms of dementing diseases as "the natural effects of aging," while some victims are skillful at covering for themselves by playing down the impact of the early stages of their illnesses and, in general, helping themselves and their families to deny what they are all going through. Uninformed professionals and families in denial can conspire to keep the fundamental question, "What are we dealing with here?" waiting a long time for an answer—often, too long for the family and the patient to work out together the best ways of living with a dementing disease.

When questions about diagnosis are finally resolved, patients and families face new but equally urgent questions. What's going to happen from here on? When will it happen? How long will Mom be able to drive and to manage her own checkbook? How long can Dad continue to live independently, or to make decisions about his own health care? How long will my husband even recognize the people he has loved all his life? Is there any chance of slowing or maybe stopping the terrible destructiveness of the disease? What can medicine really do to help? Can those of us who love this person do anything? What resources are there in my community?

But when Barbara Johnson stands before her sleeping father she needs a different kind of help. She needs *moral* help. She's struggling to understand what exactly she's doing when she tells him the truth, how far she has to go to keep her promises, what adult children owe their frail and aging parents, what marriage is supposed to mean in sickness and in health, and what counts as a loving response from the rest of the family to those who do the hands-on care. All of these problems are moral ones, because they have to do with what's *right* to do, with how one *ought* to behave. And they all require active (even if temporary) solutions.

But Barbara's struggling with something else, too—something that's even harder than the solvable problems that are on her mind. She's struggling with how to live in the face of the problems she *can't* solve. And this is really the heart of the moral task that confronts her: to keep herself whole as she meets the challenge of her father's illness, without crumpling under the weight of it, without becoming hard and embittered, without protecting herself by turning away from her father's need. She has to figure out how to be faithful to her ongoing moral commitments and how to form the new ones that may be required. She has to know the difference between what can be helped and what can't, and she has to be able to revise her judgments as the disease progresses. She has to try to stand fast. For all of us, that is perhaps the most deeply moral activity. For those who have undertaken the care of a person with a dementing disease, it is also perhaps the most difficult.

This book is for Barbara and others who are struggling to be, feel, and do what is loving and responsible as they care for family members suffering from dementing diseases. It consists of stories—one to a chapter—we have created to describe what a particular family might be going through at a particular point in the progression of a dementing disease. None of the characters is intended to resemble anyone we know or have heard of, but their experiences are based on real-life stories told to us by over two dozen family caregivers, who are themselves grappling with the issues we raise here.

Stories—whether true or fictional—are always told by selecting certain details out of the vast array life lays before us, and arranging them in a way that makes sense. The stories in this book are no exception. They are told in an attempt to make sense of a crucial job families perform for their ill and, finally, dying loved ones. To make sense of that activity, however, we had to do more than *acknowledge and describe* what the Barbaras of this world are going through. We had to offer ways of *understanding* it—ideas that might be of use to busy, distressed, and sometimes exhausted caregivers who have neither the time nor the energy to sort out all these things on their own. We spent a number of years at the Hastings Center—a research institute devoted to ethical issues in medicine—thinking about what the work of caregiving means in the context of family life. In these stories, we have combined our experience as researchers with the experiences of family members who are caring for loved ones with dementia.

A word about how we use pronouns. We've tried to avoid using "he" to mean either a man or a woman. When we make a general point, we usually use "they." Where this is clumsy, we tend to use "she" in chapters where the patient is a woman, and "he" where the patient is a man.

Getting Moral Help

Family members involved in the care of a person suffering from progressive dementia may have friends, relatives, clergy, or a support group with whom they can talk over their problems—both those that must be solved and those that can't be solved—but they will find that little has been written about the most morally troubling issues of family caregiving. This book will address those problems. Here, we help people like Barbara to anticipate and carefully think through a number of the ethical concerns that surround dementing diseases, so that the anguish they *must* feel is not made worse by anguish that is *avoidable*.

In this book, we try to identify in detail the moral tasks that face family caregivers, and we offer suggestions for better ways of coping with them. But, you may ask, aren't moral tasks just the ones about which people always say, "There are no right or wrong ways to do them"? Don't they involve the most personal and individual decisions possible? Indeed they do, but that doesn't mean there are no right or wrong ways to do them, and it doesn't mean that nothing is gained by learning how others have done them.

Our moral commitments reflect something very basic about us, about who we take ourselves to be, and about our deepest hopes for ourselves, those we live with, and our world. In this respect, they are extremely individual and personal. At the same time, people's commitments are influenced by how they understand certain facts: what their options are, what ideas undergird them, and where their priorities lie. People are also influenced by other people, both those in their families and those outside them. These others will also have moral commitments that reflect *their* understanding of the options, *their* grasp of the ideas, and *their* sense of the priorities. Disagreements are possible about all these matters, but so is conversation, persuasion, give-and-take, and compromise that needn't take away anyone's integrity.

It's tempting to think that people caring for someone with a dementing disease have enough problems without having to worry about the moral niceties. Yet, just as with dementia itself, closing one's eyes to these problems won't make them disappear. We believe that they will trouble most if not all family caregivers. Our aim, then, is to provide practical, solid help to those who are thinking through and living with the ethical challenges of caring for relatives with Alzheimer's or similar diseases.

PROBLEMS TO BE SOLVED

The larger task of living through this difficult period involves solving the smaller moral problems not once but repeatedly. What was at first an adequate response can become less so as the dementia progresses, and new strategies must be found.

Family caregivers routinely have to worry about telling the truth, keeping promises, coming to grips with the meaning of serious illness, preserving the patient's dignity, and maintaining familial relationships, although they may not use the words *moral* or *ethical* to describe their problems (we'll use those words interchangeably). Some of these problems arise as dementia challenges a family's ability to care not only for the patient's body, but for something deeper, something more like the patient's "true" self. Other problems have to do with tradeoffs among competing values: the patient's safety versus the patient's independence, for example, or the familiarity of home versus the reliability of institutional care. And a final set of problems has to do with conflicts within the family—differences of opinion about what kind of care is appropriate, or the competing claims of children or spouse on the caregiver's energy and attention. The moral problems Barbara must face and must solve—sometimes repeatedly—include these:

- **How can I honor my father's dignity when he acts in ways that embarrass him or me?**

"Dignity" is a more complicated idea than we sometimes realize. When we speak of dignity, we often have two different senses of the word in mind, one having to do with *what we are* and the other with *what we can do*. The first sense reflects our feeling that we all have a certain worth—a dignity that ought to be respected by others—simply because we are people. We aren't just objects for other people to use. Dignity, however, also seems to concern our ability to do things, particularly to control our own lives in ways that are appropriate to our circumstances. Dignity in this second sense recalls the word's original Latin meaning, "fitting" or "suitable": we are meant to behave in ways that are suited to our age, gender, occupation, or social standing.

As Barbara knows all too well, a dementing disease can often involve both lapses and outbursts that seem to lessen the patient's dignity and cause embarrassment to him and those who love him. Early in his illness, her dad was deeply ashamed of forgetting people's names, and of the occasional lapses in his conversation. A very sociable person all his life, he dropped his friends like hot coals rather than suffer the indignity of having them drop him. Barbara felt that the loss of his friends was one of the worst things the disease did to him, but she didn't know what to do about his fear of losing his dignity in the eyes of his friends. Nor was she sure how she should deal with the things he did that were inappropriate to his age and social standing (and in that sense undignified) without taking away his dignity as a person.

- **How can I help Dad keep a sense of himself as someone who is more than simply the victim of a dementing illness?**

Having a dementing disease is a central fact in a person's life. But people are more than their diseases, and as the person's own ability to express who he is through his words and actions fades, preserving his identity becomes more and more the job of those who love and care for him. Think of what you do to a person with Alzheimer's disease when you introduce him to someone by saying, "This is Henry. Henry was a lawyer." One man who was introduced this way gently interrupted: "I *am* a lawyer." This man was fighting to maintain his sense of self—an extremely precious thing—against the incursions of his disease. Those around him missed an opportunity to be his ally in this struggle.

• How can I help my father plan for his future—a future in which decisions must be made about financial matters, medical treatment, and other issues that affect not only the person who is ill but also those whose lives are intertwined with his?

What about a "living will," or some other form of advance planning for a time when life-sustaining treatment might not be wanted? How would Barbara's dad feel about tube-feeding if he couldn't swallow anymore? And how will he and Barbara both feel if she can't continue to take care of him? How will they feel if he has to go to a nursing home?

As with any illness, managing a dementing disease involves making many decisions. These decisions are both extremely difficult and extremely important, concerning everything from how and where a person will live, to how and when death will occur. The person most affected by the decisions—the one who is ill—is less and less able to understand what is at stake, less able to form an opinion about what should be done, and less able to express that opinion, even supposing he had formed one. Barbara's father has now passed the point of being able to do any of these things—but Barbara talked to him when he still could. It was crucially important to consult him then, not only because it was his care and his life that were under discussion, but also because good advance planning was needed to relieve burdened family members of at least part of their load of grief and guilt.

• How can I give, or help my father get, the kind of care he needs right now?

Barbara needs to make sure her dad is bathed, fed, taken to the toilet; that his personal appearance is cared for. Further, she needs to ensure his physical safety while preserving such independence as he can manage. Simply finding out how to get the help that Barbara's community makes available to demented persons and their families has been a difficult responsibility for her. But whether hands-on care is provided by helpers from the community, by family members, by professionals the family has hired, or any combination of these, there remains the problem of knowing how to adjust care to the real needs of the person who is ill. Proper care for his physical well-being might require relinquishing some degree of independence in the interests of safety. Yet proper care for his dignity, for his sense of himself as a person, may require exactly the opposite tradeoff.

• **Is it ever all right to lie to demented people? Can I lie and still deserve the trust of someone who is suffering in this way? Is lying always disrespectful?**

Almost everybody, at some point in life, will avoid uncomfortable truths, "edit" their own memories, mislead others, and even sometimes tell out-and-out falsehoods. And almost everybody feels uncomfortable about lying repeatedly. As Barbara wrestles with this problem, she has put herself in her dad's shoes and acknowledged that *she* would feel very uncomfortable if it turned out that someone was lying to *her*. Even so, she also knows from experience that the price of avoiding a lie can sometimes be just as high as the price of telling one.

While people will agree that one ought to tell the truth whenever possible, it's not so easy to say precisely why that's so. To understand better whether and when it's morally okay to break the rule against lying, it's necessary to figure out just what's at stake in telling the truth or failing to do so. Once family caregivers have figured this out for a given situation, it's easier for them to see what to do.

• **What should I do if Dad asks me to help him kill himself so he can escape the worst of the disease?**

More even than the physical suffering that may accompany old age and death, many people fear the long, slow decline of their mental abilities. Pain can be alleviated with analgesics and met with a kind of noble courage; human relationships can often be maintained even if someone is suffering greatly. But dementia is different. There is no painkiller to make it go away, and in the end it takes from us even our ability to recognize those with whom we have built our lives, even our ability to recognize ourselves. In the face of this, it's no wonder that suicide appears an acceptable—perhaps attractive—option to many people. The first person Dr. Jack Kevorkian helped with his suicide machine, Janet Adkins, turned to him because she preferred death to dementia.

What should families do in the face of a loved one's desire to die? Is there anything that can be done to provide a demented person with alternatives that are attractive enough to make suicide seem undesirable? Can we, for example, distinguish between his progressive dementia, which is not curable, and his depression, which may be? Can we persuade the person that he can't lose his dignity no matter what the disease does to him? And if all attempts to safeguard the dignity of the demented person and all efforts to improve his situation fail, can we in good conscience help this person die? Can we live with ourselves if we *don't* help? How can we reconcile what suffering members of our families need from us with what we owe our consciences and the wider communities of which we are all a part?

• **How can I balance what I owe to my own children and my spouse against the increasingly heavy burden of caring for my demented father?**

As if walking one tightrope at a time isn't hard enough, family caregivers have to walk a number of them all at once. They must skillfully weigh the conflicting needs and interests of the person who is ill, but they also have to respond to the needs, desires, interests, and claims of other family members.

Barbara's husband didn't feel she was doing a good job of this. If you asked him, he would say he left because Barbara's devotion to her father was eating up so much of her time and attention that it effectively ended their relationship. He believes she showed by the choices she made that her marriage wasn't very important to her. Barbara herself, of course, looks at it differently: she thinks George kept his promise to be faithful "for better," but lacked the integrity to hang in there "for worse." Regardless of who is right, there are times when she feels not only angry at her husband for letting her down but angry at herself for allowing so much of her life to be consumed by her father's care.

What do we owe our children or our spouses, and how stringent are those obligations? And how should we resolve disagreements among family members about sharing the burdens of care? Just as it's important to talk with the person facing dementia about his future care, so too is it important for family members to talk among themselves about how to divide the tasks of care. Many important differences and old resentments are apt to surface when families get together and talk about which people are and which aren't doing their share, so these conversations can be dangerous. What can be done to make them productive rather than damaging?

• How can I take care of myself when I'm· so busy responding to everyone else's needs?

It sometimes seems as if caregiving is a zero-sum game in which those who get the care take away from those who give it, leaving the caregiver empty and drained. Part of the balancing act is to make sure caregivers include themselves in the care they give others. How can they do this without being selfish? Where's the finc line between taking one's own needs and interests too seriously and not taking them seriously enough?

In the course of caring for her dad, Barbara discovered something that other people in her situation have noticed too: providing intensive amounts of care for someone else can enlarge your capacity to care. It can change your priorities, make certain things seem trivial that used to matter a great deal, increase your sense of the ill person's importance and value. It can make you a stronger and better person. It can also, of course, leave you irritable and mean-spirited.

What personal resources can caregivers muster to meet the demands of life more gracefully? What habits of character can they cultivate that will allow them to avoid feeling constantly angry and resentful, or hopeless and overwhelmed? And how does the progression of the dementing disease prompt caregivers to alter their strategies for self-care as time goes on?

• **When the demented person is not my parent but my spouse, how does this change the kind or quality of the care I give, and how does giving this care change me?**

Ordinarily, different people in the family will need different amounts of familial care. If needs are equal and in conflict, who gets what? Should our ill spouses win out over our children? Should parents lose out to ill husbands or wives? Should you encourage your children to help you with your spouse's care, even if they have small children of their own? And even if we are able to answer these questions, how can we tell if needs are "equal" or not?

• How can family members resolve, or at least live with, disagreements over who will give care, the type of care, and how much it will cost?

Different family members see things differently. They often disagree about how much direct involvement in the care of a relative is necessary or desirable, and these disagreements can damage what once were loving relationships. What Barbara's dad really needed, for instance, and even how sick he was, became matters about which Barbara and her former husband very definitely didn't see eye to eye. And as if that weren't bad enough, Barbara's older brother, Bob, also thought she often overstated how sick Dad was. Such differences can lead to serious problems within the family. Some of these disagreements will come out of long-standing interpersonal issues—for example, the resentment Bob felt because Barbara was Dad's favorite child. Other disagreements arise when family members come to terms with dementia at different speeds and in different ways.

Regardless of their origin, however, these differences can become moral differences. People have different ideas about what adult children in general owe their parents, and even more, about what specific children owe their parents. When Barbara presses her brothers for more help, she runs into both these problems. Rick says she's foolish to spend so much of her life caring for Dad now that he really can't tell whether he's living at home or in a long-term care facility, while Bob nurses the aforementioned grudge, saying that since Dad never had any time for him when he was a kid, he's not going out of his way to help him now. For her part, Barbara feels exploited by both these attitudes, and her relationship with her siblings has gotten pretty rocky. She is becoming more and more isolated from her family as well as her friends.

The tasks involved in caring for demented people are burdensome enough without costing caregivers some of their most precious possessions— good relationships with people they have known and loved all their lives. Yet it can be terribly hard to discuss such difficult matters in ways that are productive, practical, and healing, rather than divisive.

• How can I keep my memories of Dad in happier days from being blotted out by how he looks and acts now?

Dementia takes away the ill person's past as it erases the memories that meant so much to him, that are so much a part of who he is. It also takes away his future, foreshortening life and destroying anticipation. These losses threaten not only the person with the disease but also those who love and care for him. The weight of caregiving may be so great and the changes so deep that a loving spouse or child loses sight of the person being cared for. Not only can the incessant demands of the day interfere with one's ability to see past the patient's needs to his *current,* still valuable self but that neediness can make it difficult to keep a vivid sense of who he *used to be,* and of how things were in the good times. When the past slips away, it takes with it a future in which these memories might continue to console and enrich us.

Barbara has struggled to hold on to her image of her father. She always saw him as a somewhat shy, soft-spoken man who seemed at the same time trustworthy, loving, strong, and essentially independent. Now he has become loud, sometimes vulgar, self-centered, and essentially dependent on her. Remembering her dad as he was has not been easy, and as that memory slips away, she is sometimes furious that she's been trapped into doing so much for a nasty stranger. And then, of course, she feels very guilty about her anger. How can she better come to terms with these feelings? What are the beliefs—about her dad, about her duties, about herself and the rest of the family—that go hand in hand with her feelings?

WHEN THE PROBLEMS CAN'T BE SOLVED

How tough is a human self, and how bad do things have to be for a caregiver before she begins to disintegrate? When we enter the world as infants, our personalities are fluid, open to being shaped by all kinds of social forces, including, most importantly, our interactions and relationships with the people who are nearest to us. The basic structures of our personalities become set in late childhood, perhaps around the age of eight or ten, by which time we have acquired defense mechanisms, a set of strategies for dealing with people, and a sense of our own identity. Our adult lives are spent refining, rather than radically altering, the person who emerges from childhood.

As we continue to interact with the world, our personalities generally remain stable, but while they may be relatively tough, they are far from immune to the blows of illness or misfortune. When those blows are inflicted repeatedly and the person lacks adequate social and emotional support, her identity begins to crumble around the edges. In extreme cases, as when a person is held hostage by terrorists or undergoes sustained torture, her personality can even shatter. If, as folk wisdom has it, suffering builds character, it is also true that too much suffering damages it. As Barbara pulls her robe more tightly about her in the early morning light, she is expressing a very real need to hold herself together during this difficult time in her life.

What will she have to do if she is to keep herself from crumbling, or becoming embittered, or retreating into indifference? Many things, not the least of which is cultivating courage and a sense of humor. But in this book we are going to pay close attention to three tasks in particular that have a special moral force. The first is staying true to oneself. The second is accepting gracefully what can't be changed. The third is seeing things clearly.

Staying true to yourself is a way of protecting your moral center—that core of values, beliefs, and commitments that are *your* way of being in the world. It's a kind of moral steadiness, which allows others to depend on you, not only on a day-to-day basis or in the long run, but also when—as in Barbara's case—push comes to shove and your ability to rise to the occasion is put to the test. Being true to yourself doesn't mean you won't have lapses—occasional outbursts of bad temper, carelessness, or egotism. It *does* mean that you don't lose sight of who you are. You keep your central values, beliefs, and commitments from shriveling up or seeping away.

Standing fast allows you to resist the twin temptations of avoidance and denial. For many of us, becoming demented is our worst nightmare—just barely edging out the fear that it might happen to someone we dearly love. We avoid what we fear, and fear feeds denial. However silly it may sound, all of us are capable of supposing that if we pretend something very disagreeable isn't there, it might just go away. Denial of dementia is all the more tempting because the symptoms that show up first aren't easy to distinguish from the common stereotypes of old age. For the longest time Barbara, her dad, and the rest of the family took refuge in the fact that Mr. Kessler had always been a little absentminded. "Everyone forgets," after all, and "it's only natural to grow a little vague as you get on in years." For months everyone in the family repeated these phrases as if they were magic.

While such denial can be an important psychological coping mechanism, it also lets us avoid responding to another person's very real needs. For Barbara this avoidance was only temporary, but for her husband it was more than that. If Barbara's judgment of him is correct, he let some core commitments slip away. He didn't stand fast. From one's own perspective, letting go of core commitments amounts to betraying something important about oneself. From the perspective of others, it means one can't be trusted. That's how Barbara's husband seemed to her.

If staying true to yourself is like courage in that it gives you the strength to do what must be done, accepting what you can't change is something like a sense of humor: it's an attitude that helps when nothing *can* be done. It's a quiet daily going on unhampered by fantasies of fixing everything or making up for it all somehow.

This kind of acceptance isn't the same as hands-in-your-lap resignation—it's not a passive enduring. It's just the opposite. It takes an active, continually revised understanding of what must now be. This kind of acceptance is what keeps us from a self-glorifying but useless martyrdom. It lets us see the limits not only of what can be done but of what *we* can do.

For Barbara, the struggle to accept gracefully what she couldn't change began with a whole lot of useless regret. Why hadn't she taken that trip with Dad ten years ago, when he was still in good health? Why had she been so impatient with him when she was going through her divorce? And for that matter, if she had only been kinder and more attentive to her husband when she first started caring for her father, maybe things would have worked out differently and she'd still be married. "What if?" "If only," and "It might have been" ran round and round in a continual refrain as she tried to come to terms with the damage her father's illness had inflicted on her own life. What Barbara had to learn was a different, less self-absorbed way of being.

Standing fast and graceful acceptance both depend on seeing clearly. It is clear-eyed perception that allows you to see not only when and how to respond but also the limits to response. It's the ability to grasp the seriousness of what you have to deal with, a capacity for estimating repairs, a shrewdness about your own strengths and weaknesses. It's a way of paying attention.

Her ability to see clearly is what allows Barbara to hold fast to her commitments, her values, her attitudes—central features of her moral identity. The shrewdness that keeps her from fooling herself, that puts the brakes on wishful thinking or self-indulgence, is what made it possible for her to let go of the idea that her dad was just becoming a little forgetful, which in turn permitted her to start meeting his needs rather than avoiding them. Likewise, her ability to see that she is not a superwoman helped her to stop scrambling repeatedly through vain regrets. The insight that she's just Barbara, warts and all, led her to understand that she doesn't have to be so sorry she didn't do everything just right, and she doesn't have to be perfect now.

1

Coping with the Early Stages

MARY O'KEEFE is fifty-seven, but she could easily pass for ten years younger. After spending her youth and her early middle age as a full-time homemaker, she's devoted the last decade to becoming a professional caterer—a lifelong ambition. She takes a deep satisfaction in being able to express herself through her cooking and prizes her independence even more than she thought she would, especially since catering has finally started to pay her a reasonably comfortable income.

One helping of love for what you do combined with a dollop of personal pride turned out to be a good recipe for staying vigorous and fresh. Ms. O'Keefe has been through a lot in her life—a nasty divorce and a bout with breast cancer—but lately she's been relaxed, confident, and successful, and the people closest to her have tended to smile when they think about how nicely her life has come together.

That's why it wasn't just devastating but also painfully ironic when the symptoms started showing up. Ms. O'Keefe rattled her daughter Janet when she put the mail in the refrigerator one day. And because it was so completely out of character, she worried her friends when she began to be late for appointments because she somehow lost her way.

But if her friends thought these episodes were cause for concern, Ms. O'Keefe thought they were horrifying and absolutely intolerable. She couldn't stand the embarrassment. Besides, she didn't want her "lapses" to upset her friends and acquaintances any more than they already had. So quietly that most of them failed to notice at first, she began to turn down their invitations and to spend more and more time at home. She simplified her catering menus and started finding reasons to refuse jobs. In short, she began to cut the ties that connected her to the life she loved.

She couldn't, however, avoid Janet, who had been living with her mother since her own recent divorce. But she's done her best to avoid situations in which Janet might have to "make allowances" for her. Unfortunately and inevitably, her best hasn't been quite good enough, and Janet has had to make adjustments to the changes in her mother's abilities. Things have now reached the point where these allowances and excuses are becoming second nature to Janet—so much so, in fact, that most of the time she hardly notices she's making them. For the last several months Janet's convinced herself (almost) that there isn't anything really so odd about Mom's behavior. She firmly believes this—except perhaps late at night, when she wakes, worries, and finds it hard to go back to sleep.

As Ms. O'Keefe has less and less to do with people outside her home, she grows more and more dependent on Janet to fulfill her needs for companionship. Janet too is seeing less of her friends. She's not as likely to go out in the evenings. Even long-distance phone calls with her sister Pam and her brother Nicholas and their families, which used to be a weekly routine, have fallen off. Like her mother, Janet is losing some of her own connections with life. More and more often she feels as if she can't go on, and she finds herself standing in front of the window display at work staring at nothing, her mind as blank as her morning. Alzheimer's disease is starting to claim more than one victim in this home.

Our job in this chapter is to examine some of the difficulties that confront families at the onset of Alzheimer's or other dementing diseases, looking to the experiences of the O'Keefe family for examples, encouragement, good ideas, and warnings. In many ways, of course, the O'Keefes' story will be unique to them. Other families will have to deal with different problems and will have different strengths and weaknesses. But every family in this situation faces some of the same challenges the O'Keefes are facing, and it can be useful to know not only what those are, but what people have done to meet them. In particular, as we think about life with the O'Keefes, we want to look at how families make the early stages of dementia even worse than they have to be, what an admirable response for this particular family might be, and what can be done when others aren't responding so admirably.

MAKING IT WORSE

Far from being ready to accept her illness, Ms. O'Keefe tried to cover up the early changes she was going through—and her children and friends tried to follow her lead. It was well over a year before she, her family, or even her doctor were ready to put a name to what was happening. And even when she was forced to acknowledge that she was ill, she still tried to hide what was happening to her—and so to hide herself—for as long as she could.

It would be better for Ms. O'Keefe if she could be more matter-of-fact about what she's losing, more willing to assert her remaining powers, and more relaxed about her new needs. That means it would be better if those who love and live closely with her could help to create a setting in which she finds it as easy as possible to *be* matter-of-fact, assertive, and relaxed. There is a lot they are all going to have to go through, a lot they have to learn and decide, and life will be easier if they can learn, decide, and go through as much as possible together. The trouble is, everyone is shrinking from meeting the problem straight on.

For some people, uncertainty is unbearable. Facing what Ms. O'Keefe faces, people who need to know where they stand would want to do all they could to get rid of the question marks, even if that meant certain knowledge that they had an incurable and progressive disease. But for other people, the very fact that this diagnosis is so threatening makes uncertainty look pretty good in comparison. People who can't stand too much reality might be relieved if their family doctor happened not to find anything wrong. They would push away the knowledge, if they had it, that Alzheimer's disease is notoriously difficult to diagnose. This kind of person wouldn't go out of her way to consult a neurologist or geriatric psychiatrist for a second opinion. There would be an overwhelming temptation to chalk the trouble up to fatigue, or stress, or simple old age.

When Ms. O'Keefe finally did receive her diagnosis, there was nothing even remotely matter-of-fact about her response. The news signaled to her the end of everything she had built her life around and everything she had aimed it toward. Her sensitivity about her privacy, her fastidious personal habits, her relationship to her family and friends, her career as a caterer—all were in jeopardy. And she couldn't turn to her loved ones and closest friends to help her face this danger, because she felt not only a crushing sense of loss but an equally crushing sense of shame.

KEEPING UP APPEARANCES

Janet's sister Pam and brother Nicholas, along with their own spouses and children, had a hard time understanding what was happening to Ms. O'Keefe. It took them longer than it took Janet to catch on, because their mother managed to do a superb job of keeping up appearances during the quarter of an hour or so each week when they spoke with her on the phone. And because *they* didn't want anything major to be the matter either, they weren't able to take Janet's worrying seriously for quite a long time. This, of course, made Janet feel there must be something wrong with *her* if she could be imagining such a frightening illness for her own mother.

Getting a reasonably firm diagnosis at this point could actually have helped Janet, because she wouldn't have felt so isolated from Pam and Nicholas and their families. Instead, she tried to keep telling herself she was just being an alarmist. She scolded herself for being too impatient with her mom, for exaggerating every little lapse, for being hypercritical. And then, of course, she stopped being "hypercritical" by trying not to notice, and that became easier the longer she pretended. So Janet too was keeping up appearances. It became a game that everyone in the family could play.

COOPERATING WITH DEMENTIA

Although Ms. O'Keefe is so humiliated and embarrassed by her illness that she pretends nothing is wrong, there is no reason for her to feel ashamed. And it's certainly not sensible for her to shrink away from the most important aspects of her life. Her strategies—not thinking about it and keeping up appearances—are actually denying her the very things she fears the disease will take away later. Cooperating with the disease in this way is becoming completely self-defeating.

It's just as unreasonable—and self-defeating—for Janet to go along with this pattern of denial and withdrawal. For months, she's used up a lot of energy trying to beat down the gnawing feeling that something is badly wrong, and in the process she is neither giving nor getting as much help as she could. Mother and daughter together are settling into a pattern that makes every day a burden. Worse still, they are doing their best to guarantee an unbearable future.

In pointing this out, we don't mean to be hard on Ms. O'Keefe, Janet, or the rest of the family. Only someone with no imagination could fail to sympathize with the O'Keefes' barrage of conflicting feelings or their temptation to bury their heads in the sand. Nevertheless, this is an absolutely crucial turning point in their shared life. For now, Ms. O'Keefe retains the mental ability to understand what is happening to her. If she has any desire to help her family respond to her illness in the way she thinks is most fitting, she had better do it while she still can.

There's still time for her to help Janet and the rest of the family work out a better understanding of what is likely to happen, what help she will need, and what role they can play in getting that help to her. Even more important, there's still time to help the family begin as they ought to go on— namely, to think of their mother not just as a burdensome responsibility, but as a *person* who has her own thoughts and feelings, her own ideas about the overall shape she wants her life to take. But because Ms. O'Keefe is pretending nothing's wrong, she's denying herself an important capacity her illness hasn't touched yet—the capacity to participate actively in plans for her future.

Janet and the rest of the family, for their part, could be helping their mother with the very difficult job of accepting the changes in her life, so that she might respond to her last illness with the courage and dignity she's always displayed in hard times. They could also be helping each other in this task of acceptance. They could be getting as clear as possible about just what problems are looming ahead, what Mom wants done about them, and what they, individually and as a family, feel they can do to meet her needs. These are things they all have the mental ability to do. But in order to start doing anything, they first have to stop cooperating with the dementia.

For a while, it didn't look as if either Mary O'Keefe or her family would be able to stop doing that. Helping one another to face the future requires the whole family to talk about what's happening, but this requirement crashes right into the wall of silence that Ms. O'Keefe and her loved ones have built around her illness. People can be very ingenious at denying to themselves what everyone else knows to be true. Denial can be a useful, even unavoidable coping device. It gives people a chance to protect their own sense of self as they gradually absorb the implications of bad news. But denial also carries real dangers, because trying not to know about a disaster often makes things much worse.

AN ADMIRABLE RESPONSE

How can people get through denial soon enough to respond constructively to a new situation?

Working through denial can be helped by professional counselors, and if a family is in a position to get this kind of help, they should consider doing it. But denial—at least the kind Ms. O'Keefe is experiencing—has ethical as well as psychological elements, and we want to explore some of these here.

SHAME

Why is Ms. O'Keefe ashamed of herself? Feeling shame involves believing that you have done something for which you can be blamed. But surely, no reasonable person could think that Ms. O'Keefe's dementia is in any sense her fault.

Unfortunately, what we actually *believe* and what we can give *good reasons for believing* aren't always the same. The shame Ms. O'Keefe feels comes out of a pretty realistic notion of how her family and friends will react when they learn about her dementia. What she really dreads, perhaps as much as anything else that may happen to her, is that they will push her outside the circle. Inside the circle is the place for "us"—we who are lucky enough to be healthy and normal, at least for the moment. Outside is the place for "them"—those who are not healthy, not normal, and therefore not really a part of things. Very important things, like the community, the family, "life."

There is nothing crazy about Ms. O'Keefe's fear. To a greater or lesser degree, many of her friends and loved ones will think, feel, and act exactly the way she's afraid they will. But the *shame* comes from the fact that Ms. O'Keefe *herself* believes she is no longer "us" but "them." This belief is damaging and it can't be justified. It can also be hard to get rid of.

Sad though it is, when a person is seen as "abnormal"—particularly if the abnormality has to do with memory or intelligence—many of us become very uncomfortable and want to avoid that person. Even sadder, the person who is uncomfortable and the person who is "abnormal" can—like Ms. O'Keefe—be the same person. This discomfort is perfectly natural. It isn't something that Ms. O'Keefe has purposely set out to feel, after all. But it is important to see that a moral judgment is playing an important role in this feeling. At some level, Ms. O'Keefe believes that ill people really are somehow made less important, less worthy, by their physical or mental limitations. They suffer a loss of status, a lessening of their dignity.

Human beings are complicated creatures, and many other beliefs may be compounding the one that says the sick are less worthy. For example, many of us have the totally mistaken but deeprooted belief that if you avoid a person with dementia, you can lower the odds that you too will end up that way. Avoiding the person who is ill makes her feel even more unworthy, even more unlovable and isolated. Everyone in the family—

including the person with the dementia—needs to be aware that such shaming and avoidance can happen. They need to hang on to the knowledge that the disease does not make the sick person less worthy of love and respect, nor does it justify turning the person into a moral outcast.

Janet didn't have access to a professional counselor at this point; she couldn't afford it for herself, and getting her depressed mother into a therapist's office was more than Janet could handle. What she did have was the ability to examine her own feelings. She first learned how to do this when she was taking acting lessons, and she's had a lot of practice since then. Even so, it was tough for Janet to admit to herself that one of the reasons she was helping her mother avoid the truth was that she was ashamed to see this woman she loved and respected turn into "a senile old lady."

Once she admitted that, she no longer needed to hold on to the beliefs that were making her ashamed of her mother. You can't always keep nasty ideas from flying into your head, but, as Martin Luther once said, you don't have to let them build nests in your hair. So Janet started to act in ways that expressed the attitude she wanted to have. She behaved as though her mother's condition was nothing to be ashamed of, and little by little she found that the unwanted beliefs had less influence over her feelings. Janet's taking the lead in this way helped both Ms. O'Keefe and the rest of the family recognize and begin to overcome their own sense of shame.

FEAR

Shame wasn't the only emotion the family had to overcome if they were to respond admirably to Ms. O'Keefe's illness. Fear is another powerful emotion, and it too can feed denial. While shame about dementia is based on beliefs that most of us would be hard-pressed to defend, fear makes much more sense. Ms. O'Keefe believed that she had a lot to be afraid of, and she was right. However, denial and avoidance, if they are at all prolonged, not only *add* to the list of problems people have to fear, but reduce the resources they have for dealing with those problems. Our very fear of dementia is, indeed, one of the things about it we most have to fear, because it can get in the way of creative and imaginative responses.

Fear can also get in the way of some very practical and straightforward responses. Medical treatment can, for example, sometimes clear up temporary dementias and minimize the symptoms of other conditions that often coexist with progressive dementias. Diseases like Alzheimer's are frequently accompanied by other mental and emotional problems, such as hallucination or depression, that can be successfully treated. The de-

mentia itself may be made worse by physical conditions—for example, not having enough to eat or
drink—that doctors can diagnose and do something about.

Fear is treacherous from a practical point of
view because it delays people from getting help.
Victims of dementia and those who care for them
are in for the duration, and it is foolish to make
life harder in the long run for what are often illu-
sory advantages up front. But aside from this practical point, fear is also *morally* treacherous, because it produces lies and deceitful evasion. As a
general rule, it's wrong to lie, because it's manipu-
lative and disrespectful and puts the person being
lied to at an unfair disadvantage. It takes away
that person's freedom.

There are other opinions about lying, of course.
Some people have even argued that the most moral
thing to do is to deceive dementia patients about
their diagnoses. A few years ago, Dr. George Markle, a physician from New Mexico, wrote a let-
ter to the *New England Journal of Medicine*
(11 March 1993) concerning his wife's death from
Alzheimer's disease:

> When it became clear that my wife had Alzheimer's
> disease, I decided to tell her that she had a condition
> of forgetfulness and that she was no more to blame
> than a person with heart disease or arthritis. I
> shielded her from television programs and articles

that discussed her dismal future. While still rational, she went along with making a living will and giving me power of attorney because I did the same at the same time for her. There was therefore no reason to cause her to suffer the dreadful anticipation that she would otherwise have had to bear.

Dr. Markle went on to say that there was no medical reason for his wife to know her diagnosis. If she'd had cancer, she would have had to be told so that she could cooperate with her treatment, but since there is nothing that could have been done to stop her Alzheimer's disease, there was no point in telling her she had it.

Dr. Markle is fairly representative of people who think it's kinder not to tell the truth to those who are ill with a dementing disease, since medicine has nothing to offer them. But this is a mistake. As we have been trying to show, there is much that *can* be done, medically and morally, to help these people and their families. Besides, there's a real question as to whether the strategy that Dr. Markle tried with his wife can succeed. It would never have worked with Ms. O'Keefe, who had already seen the television shows and read the magazine articles, and who knew full well what she was afraid and ashamed of. It's likely, of course, that Ms. Markle had seen them too. If so, her husband's attempt to shield her would have been the very thing that prevented her from receiving the comfort she could otherwise have gotten. It would have prevented her from putting a name to what she feared and from sharing her troubles with the person she loved best.

In the O'Keefe family, the real moral question wasn't so much *whether* to seek out information about the symptoms that might indicate a progressive dementia, nor whether such information should be withheld from Ms. O'Keefe or soft-pedaled; it was rather *how* she should be helped through the shame and fear that were fueling her denial, and how information about her diagnosis and prognosis should be shared. We believe that these will be the real moral questions for many other families as well.

USING THE FAMILY'S IMAGINATION

Like many family caregivers in the midst of working out their own feelings, Janet will also be supporting and sustaining her mother: helping her to face the fact that her disease is progressive, incurable, and ultimately fatal; easing her shame and fear; covering up for her in social settings. She'll be doing a lot of this on her own, since Pam and Nicholas live far away. She will likely be learning what doctors can do, what kinds of day care facilities exist in her community, what kinds of long-term care options are available, what kind of coverage Medicare provides, and, in general, how to mediate between the person with dementia and the system.

Doing this well requires an active—and precise—imagination. For example, if you overestimate the degree of confusion the person with dementia is experiencing, you're apt to become overprotective and so threaten the patient's sense of independence and self-respect. On the other hand, if you underestimate the person's burden and sense of loss, you're apt to provide too little support and so increase the patient's isolation.

Janet felt she should also be careful about her own needs for support and connection—needs that would continue throughout her mother's illness. Being a sociable person at heart, she decided to seek out others who were facing the same problems. She hoped that a network of this kind would provide an opportunity for emotional support, for feedback, and for new solutions. It was a way, she thought, to profit from other people's imaginations. She called the Alzheimer's Association.

That's how she got to know Kathy and Dwayne Bailey. Martha Bailey, Dwayne's mom, had lived in a retirement home for several years and was fairly content there. This past year, however, it became clear that she couldn't live on her own much longer, and because Dwayne was the only one of her four children who lived nearby, he was by default the person in charge. He and Kathy cleaned out their guest bedroom, moved his mom into their home, and had been looking after her for the last six months.

"Our house was the logical place for her and we're glad she's with us," Kathy told Janet, "but Dwayne's brothers took it all so much for granted that it made Dwayne mad. He felt like they were too offhand about pushing all the responsibility for his mom onto us, just because we were close by and they weren't. And you know, when we talked to other people in our situation, we found out it's completely typical—one person in the family is the designated caregiver and everybody else drops out. But Eddie only lives an hour away, and Terry and Tom aren't that much farther. And Dwayne and I don't *want* all the responsibility."

Janet didn't either. "So what did you do?"

"I didn't. Dwayne did it. He invented something he calls the Family Huddle. He called his brothers on the phone and told them he didn't want them to take it for granted that his mom's care was up to him. He said he wants them to help him plan for her future. He wants them to make decisions with him about how to keep her active and interested in life, and about handling her money. He thinks they should figure out together when and if she'll need to be in a nursing home, and worry about her heart condition and all the rest. He was so sure they'd blow him off he nearly didn't call them, but he really didn't want us to have to handle this all by ourselves. So it seemed like it was worth a try."

"Did it work?" Janet asked.

"Mixed results," Kathy said wryly. "Eddie and Terry saw his point. They hadn't meant to duck out on helping—they just took it for granted that there wasn't anything for them to do, since she was living with us. Once Dwayne came up with some suggestions, like having Eddie get her to an elder care lawyer, having Terry spell us over Memorial Day weekend so we can go out of town, and having a Family Huddle on the phone once a month to sort out any problems that come up and make plans, they were surprisingly good about it. Dwayne has to take the initiative, but they're all on e-mail, and once he figured out how to set up a computer conference, he started scheduling one every month and they've had five in a row now."

"What about his other brother?"

"Oh well—he's being a jerk. But he was always a jerk, so at least he's consistent. He doesn't even come to see her. Says it makes him feel uncomfortable and that he's too softhearted to be able to stand it. Softhearted. Isn't that a great way to keep your caring, sensitive-guy credentials? We had to write him off, but then, we'd come close to writing them all off, and it's a good thing we didn't. Dwayne gets all the credit for being mad and doing something about it. But he didn't see why on earth one kid should have to shoulder all the worry."

Janet didn't see why either. Impressed by the Baileys' imaginative solution, she resolved to make her own attempt at a Family Huddle.

FAMILY FIGHTS

A family's task at this early stage can be very hard. There may be conflict: when some family members want to keep the diagnosis from the ill person but others don't; when, like Ms. O'Keefe, that person struggles to cover up losses and refuses to acknowledge her problem, but the family wants to break through this denial; when the person with dementia balks even at attempts to get a diagnosis; or when family members themselves move through their own denial at different rates.

The O'Keefes didn't do any better than most families at dealing with these problems. True to her resolve, Janet tried regular Family Huddles with her brother and sister. Unlike the Baileys, the O'Keefes aren't all on e-mail, but Janet found out from her telephone company how to set up a conference call and they've been having them regularly. Sometimes these conversations are emotionally exhausting for everybody. There's a tendency to revert to the kind of sniping, arguing, and putdowns the three of them used to engage in when they were kids. Nicholas gets sullen; Janet gets shrill. Pam, who's the oldest, gets unbearably bossy. Janet and Nicholas think Pam's husband doesn't treat her very well. Pam and Nicholas disapprove of a number of things Janet has done in her life. Janet and Pam are jealous of the favoritism their mother sometimes shows Nicholas. These and other undercurrents get mixed up in their discussions about their mother, not only putting the discussions in jeopardy but also putting a strain on the bonds of sisterly and brotherly love.

Just as Janet had to work hard to understand herself better and to wrestle with what she learned, so the family as a whole needs to undergo a process of self-exploration and self-education. They need to know more about their own thoughts and feelings concerning dementia—thoughts they accumulated over the years when they didn't think it would involve them directly. They need to develop a realistic view of what they will be facing in the future. They need to learn as much as they can about the resources available to them. They need to become as flexible and creative as they can.

But, as Janet has just started to realize, they need something else, too—each other. There are some practical considerations here. As the daughter who lives with their mother, Janet will, at least for the time being, have to take on the brunt of caring for her. That's a problem, because Janet was hoping to take only temporary sanctuary with her mother after the divorce. At some point she'll need her personal freedom if she's going to make new friends and trade in her dead-end job at the mall for an acting career. Pam and Nicholas have young children at home, but Janet does need them to help her as much as they can. Besides, at this stage it isn't so much the hands-on care as the *responsibility* that Janet needs to share. If she can know her brother and sister are participating in the emotional and logistical adjustments that have to be made, and that they'll stand by her when things get tougher, the illness won't be so hard to face.

Janet thinks that Pam and Nicholas need their mother too. If they detach themselves from this illness, if they let disagreements about her care serve to justify their backing off altogether, they will have lost out on a crucial opportunity to demonstrate that their relationship with their mother isn't just one of convenience and use.

This is worth thinking about for a minute. Because she was a good parent, Ms. O'Keefe provided little Pam, Nicholas, and Janet with all kinds of things, ranging from food and clothing to lessons in behavior to love. But the love she gave them when they were little wasn't like a hot meal on the table or clean laundry in the drawer—it was a *relationship,* and one the children needed to be in if they weren't going to grow up badly broken. Love has to be given as well as received: when your mom is loving you, she's teaching you to love her back. In this respect, learning to love is like learning to talk. You practice by imitating someone who knows how, and before you know it, you're in a conversation. Before Pam, Janet, and Nicholas knew it, they were in a loving relationship. They were speaking as well as hearing love, and the older they grew, the more mature their own loving became.

Loving and being loved leave you vulnerable. You're open with people you love, and that means they can hurt you far more than a stranger can. If Pam and Nicholas withdraw from their mother, not because of anything she did to deserve it but just because things are tough, they'll hurt her terribly. She's likely to feel her kids are showing that, all along, they've just been using her for the clean laundry and hot meals, that it was never really a loving relationship at all. And she'll be right. That's what Janet means when she says that Nicholas and Pam need their mother. They need her because they do love her; they aren't just in this for what they can get out of her. If ever there was a time to demonstrate their love, it is now.

So the children have a good reason to hang together even when they're furious with one another, because sharing these hard times can water and feed the whole family. Doing as much as possible together can strengthen the relationships among them, help ensure that tasks are divided fairly, and provide more clarity about the sources of their friction and disagreements. A shared commitment to seeing this through as a family is a pledge that no one will abandon the others. The disagreements will be fought out rather than walked away from, and the ones that can't be settled will be lived with.

What *Is* a Family, Anyway?

How realistic is it to think that disagreements among family members can be worked out in the way we're suggesting? Doubts about the possibility of familial teamwork are magnified by the popular idea that the family has somehow "dissolved." With divorce so prevalent, a big increase in the number of parents raising children by themselves, people living together without marriage, same-sex couples, and spousal or parental abuse so widely reported, isn't the kind of family we're talking about here—tight-knit, with everybody concerned about one another—an endangered species?

In our opinion, the family as an institution is pretty tough. It's been around since prehistoric times, which is reason enough to suppose it will last a few more years. But the form itself has altered over time—an alteration that in our part of the world has lately accelerated. It's this shape-shifting that gives rise to confusion, fear, and distrust. What does it mean to be a family nowadays? Who's out, who's in, and what follows from being in or out?

Our first idea is that families aren't defined so much by what kind of people they're made up of, as by what kind of work goes on in them. Despite what Webster's dictionary might say, not all families are "a group of individuals living under one roof and usually under one head," or "the basic unit in society having as its nucleus two or more adults living together and cooperating in care and rearing of their own or adopted children." Lots of people regard themselves as family despite the fact that they are not sharing the same residence, don't recognize anyone in particular as a "head," and are no longer (if they ever were) involved in the task of raising kids. Why do they regard themselves as family? We suggest it's because of the special jobs that are going on within their relationships.

Families—both the kinds people think of as normal and the more offbeat varieties—are places where people get a kind of intimacy that is extremely important to being socially, emotionally, and morally whole. The ongoing, committed, and long-standing relationships found in families allow them to mirror back to us a detailed and historically informed knowledge of who we are. In fact, the members of our family have a great deal to do with *making* us who we are.

Even if you can't stand your sister, then, the fact that you and she go way back and were raised inside an intimate relationship means that she's an important part of your life story. She may have drifted away in adulthood; maybe for one bitter reason or another there's no relationship left between you. But if the two of you now have a responsibility to look after a parent who is suffering from dementia (because you got the good of being loved by that parent when you were children), then it will be up to you both to rebuild your own relationship, at least to the degree that allows you to cooperate in the care of your parent. In other words, being out of the family doesn't always mean you get to stay out.

What if the person who's out of the family is the person who needs the care? Suppose, for example, she is an alcoholic mother who was at best unreliable when her son was little and now that he's grown is often abusive. Does he have a duty to stay in a loving relationship with her? Relationships take at least two people, so to the extent that the alcoholism has broken this one down, there's little the son can do about it. He certainly doesn't have the full range of duties to his mother that Janet has to hers, although if there's no one else to make arrangements for her care, common decency requires him to do it. He shouldn't allow her needs to jeopardize the well-being of his own household, but those needs do pull her a little farther back into his family.

Despite all the frictions and failures in families, people still need their connections. If people are important, then these attachments are important as well, and worth the trouble it takes to maintain them.

DOING THE FAMILY HUDDLE

Since there are good reasons for Janet, Pam, and Nicholas to work hard at staying on good terms and cooperating in their mother's care, they'll have to keep talking to one another. What might these talks be like, and what can and can't they accomplish? In outline, the idea of Dwayne Bailey's "Family Huddle" is very simple. The members of the family share concerns, pool ideas, make and revise plans, and provide support for one another. Ideally, some of these meetings are face to face, and include the person who is ill. If she is only mildly demented, she may have lost her ability to initiate long-term planning while still being capable of discussing her concerns, hopes, fears, and wishes. Such discussion would give the family useful guidance for future decision making, both in situations where a particular problem has been anticipated and in those where it hasn't. Even when something unexpected comes up, if family members have thoroughly explored things with the ill

person, they may be in a better position to understand what she would say about the matter at
hand if she were able.

Other family huddles needn't include the ill person, and needn't have everybody in the same
room. Whether over the phone or through some
medium like e-mail, such conversations can provide the rest of the family with an opportunity to
express their views without censoring themselves
for the ill person's benefit. They give people a
chance to say what they are prepared to do and
what they are not prepared to do. Over time, as
the full dimensions of the problem become plainer,
such talks make it easier to see whether people's
assessments are realistic, fair to themselves, and
fair to others. This in turn allows the family to
rearrange the division of labor.

How spouses, siblings, and adult children respond to the earliest stages of the dementia may
take on a special significance that goes beyond that
moment. The way the first decisions are made,
conflicts resolved, and problems met, and the way
the family initially comes to think and feel about
the person who is ill can set patterns for what is to
come.

A big task for the family at this point will be
figuring out the best ways to share the responsibilities. Families so often simply expect that one member—usually a woman—will be the primary caretaker. The others then take less active roles,

deciding for themselves, privately, how much or how little they're going to do. This is a good way to breed resentment, ill will, and defensiveness. While in practice it's highly unlikely that tasks can always be divided equally among family members, determining just what would count as fair and what people can appropriately expect of one another is a chore that needs to be undertaken early on.

What the O'Keefes, for example, worked out was that Ms. O'Keefe and Janet would continue to live together, and Janet would do most of the day-to-day helping out. This arrangement was to continue for one year—the amount of time Janet felt she'd need to make serious plans about her own further education and career. During that period, her siblings would provide regular breaks for her. After that time, the whole situation would be reevaluated. If it turned out for the best that Janet continue to live with her mother, the others would consider themselves obliged to help her financially, perhaps contributing to her tuition or staking her to a start in business. Or maybe it would be necessary for Pam and Nicholas to help pay for a full-time caregiver.

Anyone who wants to remain in an ongoing, familial relationship, no matter how distant, with a person suffering from dementia will have to come to terms with the full impact of the disease. We've already explored the special reason why Janet, Pam, and Nicholas need to do this. But what about other family members? What about Nicholas's wife, and Pam's less-than-perfect husband? If these people wish to continue in a familial relationship with the ones caring for Ms. O'Keefe, they too have to become part of the process of providing care.

One of the reasons for this is simple fairness—to the relationship with Ms. O'Keefe, as well as to the relationships with their own spouses and with Janet. Any relationship with another person that is more than simply a matter of using her involves some readiness to take the other person's point of view seriously, on that person's own terms. If one member of the family is doing most of the hands-on work, other family members who wish to maintain a relationship with her will have to look at the situation from her perspective and respond accordingly. If they think she is doing more than is necessary, or that she exaggerates the importance of what she is doing, taking her seriously means talking things over with her to see if some agreement can be reached.

Family huddles give people a chance to explore their fears and hopes, weave a little extra solidarity into the web of family life, and carve up the tasks of caregiving. They also have a fourth function—one so important we're going to devote the next chapter to it. It's the function of visualizing the future of the person with the dementing illness—a process called *advance planning*. What people do in the future to respond to the illness will have a greater effect on the ill person than on anyone else involved. For that reason, the person should be encouraged to participate in planning that future while she can still help determine what it will be.

WHEN THE FAMILY'S RESPONSE IS LESS THAN ADMIRABLE

Ms. O'Keefe hates to think about the future, but she knows her children are working hard to help her and she wants to make things easier for them. So she did her best in the two face-to-face conversations Nicholas and Pam were able to attend. The monthly conference calls that followed the face-to-face visits were a big help to Janet, because they made her feel she wasn't having to cope with her mother's illness all by herself. As the months wore on, however, Janet began to get the distinct impression that what she'd feared earlier was indeed coming true: Nicholas and Pam were going to leave her holding the baby. Well before the year was over, there was one "good" reason after another why they had to cancel the weekends with their mother that would give Janet the breaks they'd all agreed she should have. They started talking about the possibility of a full-time caregiver, but hinted that it would be up to Janet to arrange it without any help from them. And any time she's reported to them how tired she is, or how Mom's behavior is worrying her, instead of offering sympathy and support, they've made it clear they think she should put Mom in a nursing home. But Janet doesn't agree. She sees that her mom loves her own home and feels safest there, and thinks she's perfectly capable of living there for quite a while so long as there's someone looking after her.

Let's suppose that Janet is right about this, and that Pam and Nicholas aren't living up to their responsibilities. Let's say that they are, in fact, letting everybody down. When Janet pointed this out to them, they didn't mend their ways; instead, they simply came up with fresh excuses. So it seems that Janet can't make them love their mother better, or force them to treat Janet fairly, or get them to do what's right. It looks like she's stuck.

And so she is. But she's stuck because she's remaining loyal to her mother and to her own moral commitments. In keeping faith with her mother by trying to respond lovingly and imaginatively to her illness, Janet is also keeping faith with herself. She is exercising the personal integrity that allows her mother to depend on her, and in doing so she is becoming more like the person she would ideally like to be. She is deriving quiet satisfaction from living well with herself. From that point of view, she's not so much stuck as standing fast.

Moreover, after doing everything she could to involve her brother and sister in their mother's care, Janet had the grace to stop hammering at a door that wasn't going to open. She acknowledged the limits of Nicholas's and Pam's loyalties and didn't waste valuable energy in trying to make them be other than who they were. Nor did she waste energy in dwelling on her grievances. Her opinion of her brother and sister has been lowered, but she's trying to remember that they may have difficulties she knows nothing about, and countless other calls on their time and attention.

Reacting so calmly to a situation that can be very hard for a very long time requires a clear-sightedness that's bound to desert Janet on occasion. This ability to see both what can and what can't be done, and to see where some of her own limits lie, has been the source of the grace and integrity with which she meets her mother's needs. There will be times, however, when her moral vision will fail her—when she loses her sense of humor and gets things out of proportion, when she doesn't see her mother with the eye of loving attention. But she's worked out what her overall goal has to be, and we don't think she'll lose sight of it for long: to welcome into her own life the project of looking after her mother as well as she can.

2

Making Plans
for the Future

WHEN JOSHUA CANTOR turned seventy, he lost two of the most important things in his life. One loss, the jewelry business to which he had devoted nearly forty years, was expected and regretfully planned for. It was past time to sell. Running the business had become an uphill battle against the large jewelry store chains, and profits had dropped off in the past several years even though Joshua had been putting in longer hours than when the place was in its prime. Besides, he was tired and getting on in years—he didn't need all the worry and responsibility.

The other loss was a shock. His wife, to whom he'd been happily married since he was twenty-five, died suddenly of a heart attack. She was a few years younger than he and had been so healthy and active all her life that he had always assumed she would outlive him. It wasn't until after she died that he realized how heavily he'd depended on her. Her unexpected passing shook him deeply, unseating all his hopes for a peaceful and rewarding retirement.

Mr. Cantor is now seventy-three and dealing with yet another blow. Since shortly after his wife's death, he had seemed to his family and friends somehow less able to cope with life, more absentminded, more easily confused. His children chalked up these lapses to the natural forces of grief and adjustment to widowerhood, but they also urged him to see his doctor. The doctor's examination led to repeated visits and those visits to very bad news: Mr. Cantor has Alzheimer's disease.

Like Ms. O'Keefe, Mr. Cantor and his children struggled to acknowledge and do something about the situation into which they had been thrust. Unlike the O'Keefes, however, they made good-faith efforts at first to work together as a family and try to sort out what to do. But now that Mr. Cantor and his family are starting to emerge from the shock and to confront the question of how to share the rest of their life together, a serious difference of opinion has arisen.

John, Mr. Cantor's eldest son, wants his father to transfer his assets to John's sister Anne immediately. Sheltering this money with Anne, John feels, is much better than letting a nursing home eat it up at the rate of sixty thousand dollars or more a year.

Medicare won't pay for nursing home care, but Medicaid will—as long as Mr. Cantor can prove that he owns nothing more than his house, his car, personal possessions, and a modest amount of cash. John thinks they'll have to act fast, since, to avoid penalties, the money has to have been transferred three years before a person applies for Medicaid. There's no telling how much longer Mr. Cantor will be capable of making the transfer, and no telling when he may need daily professional care.

John points out that his dad's assets aren't just money—they represent the full forty years of his life's work. It's only right that the family should do what it can to preserve that, especially since sheltering the money with Anne is perfectly legal.

"Look," he says to his dad. "The whole health care system's badly designed and unfair to people like you. It's built around high-tech, intensive, short-term treatments that are supposed to make a sick person well. It's *not* designed for people with long-term problems like Alzheimer's disease, who need lower-tech care—but for months or years—and who aren't ever going to get well. People like you get nothing while somebody who needs his second round of triple coronary bypass surgery gets a full ride. It's crazy. Why should somebody with a heart condition be covered and treated better than you? You're being discriminated against."

John is arguing as if the problem is to try, in the

face of an unresponsive and unjust social system, to pull what his father has worked for all his life out of the wreck of the disease that is slowly destroying him. While John doesn't say so out loud, he also thinks that in his best moments his father surely wouldn't want to spend all that money—money that could go to his children and his children's children—just to keep a badly demented person in a nicer nursing home for a few more months. If they help their dad stay at home until he's past caring about the amenities and then let Medicaid kick in, he'll get adequate care and they'll all have saved the money he had worked so hard to accumulate.

Mr. Cantor is, as he puts it, underwhelmed by John's plan. So is Anne, for two reasons. For one, she's afraid that if she accepts the transfer, she's also accepting John's share of the responsibility for her father's care. Anne has a little girl, a husband she's quite fond of, a room full of kindergartners she loves to teach, and she wouldn't at all mind becoming pregnant again. While she realizes that a good deal of her father's care will fall to her, she's determined that it will be a fair amount, one that she can balance with her other responsibilities. She's carefully watching all of John's moves in this discussion, afraid of the many good reasons he'll come up with for not doing too much to look after his father.

Like her brother, Anne thinks things that she

doesn't say out loud—not even to herself. In the back of her mind, though, she wonders whether John won't duck out on her when their dad's situation gets really bad. For most purposes John's pretty reliable—he came in very handy when Anne was a teenager and needed her old car fixed, for example. What's not so clear is whether he can stay involved and available for what might be years as their dad gets progressively worse and taking care of him gets progressively harder. John's a little bit like the health care system he's so busy criticizing: good for acute problems, not so hot for long-term care.

Anne also can't shake the feeling that this asset-transfer scheme is really nothing less than a move to defraud the government—which is to say, the taxpayers—since Medicaid was never designed for middle-class people. Her brother disagrees.

"I'm telling you, this is perfectly legal," he insists. "My lawyer says there's a whole new specialty called elder law that's grown up around this problem. It's got its own professional society— the Academy of Elder Law Attorneys—and somewhere around four thousand members nationwide. It's a field that didn't even exist ten years ago, but it's growing because health care costs are growing and the number of old people in this country is growing, and people are having to figure out how to deal with what's basically a new trend. Nobody's talking about breaking the law. What I'm proposing is legal."

"Okay, it's legal," Anne says, jangling her turquoise and silver bracelets irritably. "That doesn't make it ethical. The rules about who's eligible for Medicaid were made through a democratic process, don't forget, and they weren't made with this little end-run in mind. Before Pop got sick, you never had any problem with the idea that Medicaid was supposed to be available for poor people, not for people like us. If you gave it any thought at all, you were probably just thankful that your taxes weren't any higher."

"As a matter of fact, I didn't think about it. But now that I have, I honestly don't see that Pop has some kind of patriotic duty to save all his money over the next several years, just so he'll have it available to pay for a nursing home he'll probably never need."

John gets up from the sofa and goes to kneel by his father's chair. "Look, Pop. Suppose you decided tomorrow that you wanted to take a trip to Israel—to see Jerusalem again one more time while you've still got your health. You know what we'd say? We'd say, Fine, do it. Go to Jerusalem, have a good time. Maybe that's what you *do* want to do. If it is, I'm all for it. So's Anne. And if it's not immoral for you to transfer your assets to El Al, it's not immoral for you to transfer them to Anne."

On thinking it over, Anne admits that there might be something to this way of looking at it, but she's not as confident about this as John is. For one thing, transferring the money from her father to herself will make it easier to put Pop into a nursing home sooner rather than later. She's uncomfortable about this. If the only way the family can preserve his estate is to keep him at home as long as possible, then that's an incentive to keep him there, even if it means considerable extra trouble for his children and their families. On the other hand, if they already have the whole estate, then there's only Pop's own well-being to consider, and there won't be any reason to give that any more weight than the interests of other family members. Pop suddenly becomes just another contender for the family's resources. Anne doesn't particularly like the fact that she's thinking in these terms, but she is.

Mr. Cantor is "underwhelmed" for another reason. He's not much worried about whether John will be involved in his day-to-day care—he takes it for granted that he won't be. Nor is he worried about the Medicaid question. He's been a scrupulous taxpayer all his life, and the only feeling he has about the government is that it's finally time for him to get something back from it. No, what troubles Mr. Cantor is that giving up control of his assets makes him feel as though he's giving up control over himself, not to mention cutting the ties to his past. He feels as if he's cooperating with, rather than fighting, what the disease is doing to him.

This family obviously faces a number of problems, some on the surface, some buried deeper. They're disagreeing about who owes what to whom, they don't completely trust each other, and Anne in particular isn't altogether sure she trusts herself. How can good solutions to the moral problems of caregiving emerge among people so divided?

Part of the trouble here is that the Cantors all have different ideas about how we should live—about what makes life good and what should matter to us, both on a daily basis and in the larger scheme of things. Anne and John don't agree, for example, on what a good son or daughter 'should be willing to do for a parent, or what a good father should want to give his children, or what good citizens owe to their community or country. They also have different assumptions about whether being a woman automatically means you should be the caregiver, and different hopes and expectations about their own futures. Some of these differences seem to be colliding at breakneck speed.

But different ideas about how we should live often go along with other kinds of differences. We see the effect of the Cantor children's different personalities: Anne is an intense, romantic person who dresses flamboyantly, and John is more businesslike and dispassionate. Such different personal styles can raise suspicions about whether everyone is really acting in good faith. Fiscal conservatism can look, to a romantic, like greed; emotional intensity, to a reserved person, can look like unreliability. Furthermore, Anne and John give different accounts of their history as children growing up together. These differences can be the basis of disagreements, sometimes nasty ones, among family members.

WHY IS ADVANCE PLANNING A GOOD IDEA?

Advance planning might seem to run contrary to the old proverb, "Don't trouble trouble till trouble troubles you." Having disturbing talks with your relatives about difficult possibilities that *might* crop up at some time in the future sounds like a painful and pointless way to spend your time—something like arguing with your ex-spouse. Still, we think there are three good reasons for the Cantors to try to do some advance planning together.

The first reason has to do with Joshua Cantor himself. One of the most important ways competent, mature individuals express their personhood is by making their own decisions about how they will try to lead their lives. Mr. Cantor's situation has suddenly changed, and he hasn't had time to figure out how best to be himself in these new circumstances. In the process of thinking about what the disease is likely to do to him, getting a sense of the difficult decisions that have to be made, and making as many as possible while he is still able, he can examine, refine, and expand his own particular view of what the good life is for him. For many people, decisions about how to live out the last chapters of their lives present the final opportunity to tie up loose ends and to affirm the important values they have lived by. Creating opportunities for someone to have a say in these matters, even when he is ill with a dementing disease, is a way of respecting that person's dignity. It's also a way of resisting a major temptation: to treat the person as if he were a child.

Anne's in favor of discussing Pop's future with Pop. Assuming too quickly that he's too confused to do certain things may actually make him unable to do them, she thinks. And if making decisions is a way for him to express who he is, well, she wants to do right by him. She doesn't want to contribute to any sense that Pop has been demoted from his status as a dignified adult. Of course, she doesn't know for a fact that he'll be interested in making plans with her and John about his illness. However, he used to take the lead in things like helping the kids choose what college to go to or planning the family's vacations, so Anne thinks that involving him in their decision making is an expression of respect that's appropriate for him. It wouldn't have mattered as much for her mom, who never thought of herself as the person in charge of decisions. But Pop did.

The second reason why at least some advance planning should take place with everybody together—this is John's reason—is that since he and Anne are going to have to call the shots later on, they have a responsibility to try to learn what their dad needs and wants. John doesn't think it would be right to step up his dad's care when he's dying, for example, if it turns out that Pop would've hated that—and especially if he had never bothered to ask. Just as important, he thinks, is making sure that Pop knows what he and Anne are willing to go along with. For instance, if Pop thinks he's going to keep living by himself until he's bedridden, and the kids think he'll have to have supervision long before that, he needs to know that they won't honor his wish. Then they may be able to come up with a plan they all can live with.

While not all problems will be solved nor all disagreements headed off (talking about things in the open can sometimes lead to even sharper disagreements), much of the friction between patient and caregiver stems from different beliefs about what is actually happening. If agreement can be reached about that, then it can more easily be reached about what should be done in response, and about who should do it. In any case, it's worth clearing up misunderstandings based on assumptions that seem obvious to one person, but not at all obvious to anyone else.

A third, often unappreciated reason for advance planning is that people don't always *have* clear preferences about things that may be completely foreign to them. The Cantors have no previous experience with Alzheimer's disease. Do *you* know what medical treatment you'd want if at some point you were demented and in a diaper and living in a nursing home, and you came down with a life-threatening pneumonia? Most of us don't have a fully formed preference about something like that, because we don't know enough about what it would be like for us, or what the fallout would be for other people. Figuring out what we would want later on is often best done in dialogue with other concerned and involved people—the more so, as those people will surely be affected by what we want.

WHY IS ADVANCE PLANNING DANGEROUS?

"I'll tell you what makes me so nervous about talking with Pop and John about Pop's care," Anne said on the phone to a friend one day. "I'm afraid that if we disagree with each other, people's feelings will be hurt, and we might even end up on bad terms with each other."

"Well," said the friend, "at my office, people disagree with each other all the time and everything jogs along pretty smoothly anyway."

"Yeah, but that's because when you're at work you don't really care if you step on a few toes here and there. When it's your brother and you love him, you can't help caring."

"True," her friend agreed. "And your family stays in your life longer than your co-workers do. My sister is always my sister, even when she's being awful, whereas my boss is my boss only until I quit—or get fired—and go to work for someone else."

This special feature of family relationships has moral implications. You might not be willing to say what you honestly think to your brother, either because you don't want to hurt his feelings, or because you think you have to paper over your differences with him so there won't be a visible rupture in the family. This is what's going on between Anne and John. Anne is uneasy about her brother's real commitment to the project they're trying to put together. She worries that if she pushes too hard against his point of view, he may simply become disaffected, both with her and with the task of caring for Pop.

John, on the other hand, has implicit confidence in Anne's commitment; he knows that she's in it for the long haul, that she'll always be there for him when he wants her, and always be there for his dad as well. This doesn't mean that he's plotting to exploit her; fairness is a value for him, just as it is for her. It does mean that he's more comfortable with arguing vigorously for his own perspective on things. He doesn't want to hurt her feelings, of course, but he thinks that the issues they are considering are of great importance, and worth some hurt feelings if necessary. He doesn't worry that any real damage will be done.

These differences are impossible to set completely to one side. Family history, clashing moral perspectives, personal idiosyncracies, and gender stereotypes may all play a role here, and are deep and powerful forces. They can be kept from disrupting the proceedings, however, if the involved parties have a clear sense up front of what they're trying to do and of what might get in the way.

ADVANCE PLANNING: HOW TO BEGIN

"I don't understand why you're pushing this," said Anne to John the next time they stopped by Pop's house together. "I definitely don't want to take over the responsibility for handling Pop's money." She was perched on the arm of her dad's chair, and now she reached over and rumpled his hair. "I don't see the point in it, Pop. If you ever need more care than we can give you, well, John and I will work something out. Together. We'll hire somebody, or try to get creative about involving other people. Maybe we'll reach a point where you run out of money and need us to help pay your bills, but we can cross that bridge when we come to it."

"Yeah, but the time is going to come when we have to take more responsibility for you, Pop," John replied. "Not right away, of course—I don't mean that. And naturally, whatever we have to do, we'll do it together. I'm just saying that now is the time we should be protecting Pop's assets."

John tapped the table with his pen. "The best way to do that is to have him live here as long as he can and then have him move in with one of us. Either way, we'll keep him at home as long as it matters to him to be at home. We won't move you to a nursing home, Pop. Not unless you get to where you don't really care where you are—and that might never happen. But if it ever did, at least you'd have the comfort of knowing that your property is safe."

At this point, Mr. Cantor rose to his feet and left the room, shutting the door hard.

Whatever else they disagreed about, Anne and John were of one mind in seeing this as a bad start. They decided to put the money issue on the back burner for a while and start over again. Advance planning still seemed like a good idea, but they were going to have to go at it more thoughtfully.

They began by proposing that their discussions

be fairly formal. The family would set aside regular times to talk over how things were going with Mr. Cantor's illness, what needed to be done next, and what would need attention in the future. Topics unrelated to his disease wouldn't be discussed during the times set aside for Mr. Cantor.

John thought it would be a good idea to write up what happened at each meeting and to make copies for everyone. This was partly so they could keep track of what had been decided, but also to later convince doctors and other caregivers outside the family that their decisions had something of Mr. Cantor's own authority behind them. Anne agreed, so long as John was willing to rotate the note-taking task, rather than sticking her with it permanently.

Anne and John also tried to figure out who needed to be in on these discussions and who could safely be left out. Mr. Cantor did have a younger brother in California, but their lives hadn't been closely connected for a long time, and Mr. Cantor thought that just keeping George informed of what was happening would probably be enough. Furthermore, he was adamant about not involving any of his friends in these discussions. So the meetings would be held with Anne and her husband Philip, John and his wife Wendy, and John and Wendy's two teenage sons, who were close to their grandfather. That way, no one who needed to be in was left out; no one who wanted out was forced in. Other families may not, of course, be quite so lucky in these respects.

Another important point that Anne and John agreed on was that, while advance planning was a good idea, it would be impossible to foresee everything that might affect their sense of what was best, or even feasible. Their plans might have to be revised at a later date, and if they paid attention to the *reasons* behind the decisions they made now, they'd be that much better able to preserve the spirit of those decisions in the future. Therefore, the reasons would be written down along with the decisions.

Anne and John also thought about how to make the conferences hospitable enough so that people would feel they could say what they really thought. They reminded each other up front that the problem of their father's illness was a problem that everyone in the family had agreed to share equally. They acknowledged that personality differences would get in the way of complete openness and equality in their discussions, and they all agreed to try to compensate for this.

So that was the plan: Mr. Cantor and his family caregivers would meet together regularly to discuss how people were doing, to identify issues, to make new plans, and to revisit old ones. Mr. Cantor would be a part of these discussions for as long as he could. But even after he was no longer able to participate meaningfully, the family would continue to meet.

As often happens, however, the reality turned out to be a little different from the plan.

ADVANCE PLANNING: CAN WE TALK?

Advance planning sessions are supposed to help the person with the dementing illness get a sense of what decisions may need to be made and what the options are, and then to actually make some choices. Many of the choices have to do with what will happen in the future, when a person like Mr. Cantor won't be able to fully understand what's going on and what might be done about it. Some of these situations can be forecast fairly well and the planning sessions are an opportunity to do that.

Mr. Cantor had already given some thought to this sort of thing. After his wife's death, he filed a legal document called a health care proxy, which is also known as a durable power of attorney for health care decisions. This document is one form of advance directive; it appoints someone to make decisions about treatment you will or will not get, in the event that you are too ill to make these decisions for yourself. Health care proxies allow you to choose someone who will make the decisions in your place.

Other advance directives—living wills, or, more

broadly, treatment directives—contain directions not about *who* decides but about *what* decisions should be made. For instance, a person may direct that if he ever is so unfortunate as to fall into an irreversible coma, he doesn't want to be kept alive on a respirator. Or he might direct that if he is dying of an incurable cancer, he wants only comfort care. Of course, it's also possible to have "mixed" advance directives, which both name a person to make decisions and give that person specific directions about the patient's health care preferences.

In some states—like New York—living wills haven't been recognized by the legislature (which doesn't mean they wouldn't be honored in court), but people are encouraged to name a "health care agent" who will make medical decisions for them should it become necessary. The agent's power isn't unlimited, and depending where you live, there may be rather strict laws about it. For example, if you don't want to have artificially provided food and fluids under certain conditions, in some states you have to give your agent specific authorization to refuse that treatment.

Three years ago Mr. Cantor executed an advance directive in which he named his son as his agent for health care and specifically gave him authorization to make decisions about tube-feedings. However, at that time, he and John didn't really discuss what Mr. Cantor might want under various circumstances. Today, John realizes that the time to talk about it is now. If they don't, John may come to find himself in a very uncomfortable position, because he'll be expected to speak on his dad's behalf without really knowing what Mr. Cantor had in mind.

But here the Cantors ran into yet another snag. Although Mr. Cantor is perfectly capable of deciding whether he still wants John to be his health care agent, he's having considerable difficulty with his short-term memory. He forgets that he's ill with Alzheimer's disease. As a result, he's not particularly motivated to talk about his future. The whole idea leaves him cold. He hates the prospect of being so sick that other people have to do his thinking for him, and he didn't much enjoy what happened the first time John and Anne sat down to talk with him. His reluctance may also have something to do with the idea that his kids already know or should be able to figure out what he would want. Isn't that how he raised them—to take care of him in his old age and not bother him with questions?

Here, John and Anne confront what is clearly another moral problem. Should they respect their father's unwillingness to discuss the future—which would mean, of course, that they will be on their own when hard decisions need to be made? Or is it, rather, the part of a loving and judicious family to take an active role in starting the discussion?

Shouldn't they *insist* that their father pay attention to the decisions that are at hand, and do his best to give directions about them?

The answer depends on just how unwilling he is. Making good decisions for a confused person is not a trivial problem, and the burdens imposed upon the proxy decision makers are not light. In most situations similar to the one Mr. Cantor's children find themselves in, it would be both irresponsible and imprudent for the children simply to take the path of least resistance and not raise any questions at all. On the other hand, if Mr. Cantor firmly and repeatedly refuses to talk about the future, it might mean he wishes that his children would simply lift the burden of choice from his shoulders. He might be signaling that he trusts them to deal responsibly with issues he would very much rather not face himself.

There is another, even more complicated possibility. The children might be able to persuade Mr. Cantor to discuss his future, but at great cost to himself. He might be deeply disturbed and frightened by these conversations, and at a loss to understand why he is being asked to do something so intensely disagreeable. The thought of this possibility put a considerable weight on Anne and John for a time. They had to decide whether to push their father to tell them what he thought, and if they did push, how hard. They had to determine what they'd do if he continued to be unwilling to participate in planning discussions.

Anne grew so frustrated during this time that when she stopped by John's house one Saturday afternoon, it was either vent her feelings or burst. "How on earth can Pop expect us to steer blindfolded? Dammit, he has no *right* to saddle us with all the decisions that'll have to be made for him over the next few years when we have no idea what he would have wanted. We're just supposed to guess? What if we guess wrong? Honest to God, I have never seen anybody so pigheaded and downright *selfish* in all my life!"

Her sister-in-law handed her a Diet Coke while her brother propped himself against the kitchen counter, arms folded across his chest, grinning. "Getting on your wick, isn't he, Annie? I haven't seen you blow into the house like this since I let your boom box fall into the swimming pool when we were in high school. I think you're being too hard on the old man. I mean, Pop's got a *right* to make decisions about his own life, but I don't think that means he's got a *duty* to make 'em—especially since we're around to do it for him. Besides, I'm not so sure he *can* make 'em." He turned to his wife. "I didn't have a chance to tell you this yet, Wendy, but when I took Pop to the hardware store this morning he suddenly looked at me and said, 'You know, you're my favorite customer.' I said, 'Pop, I'm your son!' So he said, 'Oh well, that explains it, then.' It was all I could do not to laugh out loud."

Mr. Cantor remained reluctant to take an active role in planning his future, so his children finally regrouped. Although they felt rather peculiar about meeting without him, John, Wendy, and their two teenage boys did get together at Anne and Philip's house to discuss the situation. They decided there was no good reason to change the arrangement that had been made three years ago: John would continue to be the official proxy decision maker for his dad. But John wanted other family members—particularly his sister—to be involved in the decision making. He didn't want to do it all by himself if he didn't have to, and he also wanted to start deciding things right away. Just as he was strongly of the opinion that his dad's financial situation had to be dealt with immediately, so too he felt it was crucial that they imagine what medical and familial problems might come up, and at least sketch out potential solutions.

Anne thought it wasn't enough to anticipate problems and develop strategies on their own. She thought they also ought to let their dad know what they came up with so he could veto a decision if he wanted to. She pointed out that there was a difference between having to be involved in thinking through lots of complicated alternatives, on the one hand, and simply agreeing to or rejecting a scheme on the other. Just because Pop wouldn't participate in planning didn't mean he wouldn't want to know what they had worked out for him, or wouldn't appreciate the chance to object. At least, she argued, they should give him the opportunity to respond. And anyway, it was always possible that if they presented him with some sketched-out plans, Mr. Cantor might be willing to fill in the details himself.

John wondered if going back to him with their ideas wouldn't be hard on the old man. "Why shove possibilities down his throat when it's clear he doesn't want to deal with them? It seems to me he's already at the point where any kind of planning or organization overwhelms him, and what we're talking about here isn't just complicated, it's nasty and unpleasant. We can handle it without involving him. We lived with him long enough to know how he feels."

"Sure we did," Anne snorted. "We lived with Mom for a long time too, and we couldn't even buy her the kind of clothes she liked. Remember that suede skirt we got her for her birthday one year, and how she wore it all that day and then left it hanging in the closet? Remember how bad we felt because we'd guessed wrong? Well, what we have to guess about here is going to make us feel a whole lot worse if we don't have some sense that we're doing what he wants."

This struck Wendy, the boys, and Anne's husband Philip as a fair point, and, after some discussion, John agreed that he and his sister would let Pop know what they'd been talking about. So Anne and John did have some talks with Mr. Cantor about what they felt should be done. In the course of these talks, the older man seemed to become a little more comfortable with the subject, and responded to some of their proposals and opinions. Over time, they had the chance to talk about—and write down—his thoughts about many important things: that he didn't care so much about driving his car, for example, but he was damned if he would give up carpentry even if there was a chance he might hurt himself. And that he expected them to keep him out of the nursing home, but he also didn't want to be a burden to them. Anne toyed with the idea of taping these discussions, thinking that maybe having a record of *how* Pop said something would sometimes be as useful as a record of *what* he said. But, like a lot of interesting ideas, that one fell through the cracks.

Mr. Cantor's concerns about being a burden to them were the first things they talked about. These were followed by issues of privacy and contact with others. Like Ms. O'Keefe, Mr. Cantor had been a rather private person, but he did have several close friends. He both very much wanted to see them and very much wanted to avoid them. With the encouragement of his kids, Mr. Cantor eventually came to hope that one or two of his closest friends might be invited back into his life, and that they might even help him out with a few things that were getting beyond him.

There were many other topics the group eventually touched on. When he couldn't live by himself anymore, would he rather move in with Anne or have a home health aide? Would he like to get to know something about the activity groups and special classes that were available for people with Alzheimer's disease? Would he care to visit some local nursing homes to see if they were better than he thought?

Questions about medical care were more difficult. The family wanted to know what they should do if other medical problems came up. Having Alzheimer's doesn't, after all, protect a person from heart attacks, strokes, or cancer. If Mr. Cantor should become seriously ill, or badly injured, would he want to undergo intensive care, or would he rather just be kept comfortable, even if that meant he would die sooner? How about the kinds of medical treatment he might require because of the Alzheimer's disease itself? What did he think about being fed through a tube if the dementia progressed to the point where he couldn't eat anymore?

And then there was John's pet problem: what should be done about Mr. Cantor's money? This was very much tangled up with the question of nursing home care. Of course Mr. Cantor never wanted to go to a nursing home, but what if they

just couldn't manage to take care of him themselves? What if he started wandering away from
home and getting lost, or keeping everybody up all
night, or hitting and yelling at people? He might
be willing to have his children run his errands,
keep his checkbook balanced, dress him, and make
sure he took his pills, but how would he feel about
one of them bathing him? Giving him a bedpan?
Spoon-feeding him? Massaging him to prevent
bedsores? Changing his diaper?

ETHICAL DECISION MAKING: MORE THAN PREFERENCES

While people don't always agree about how to
make good moral decisions, nobody thinks you
can do it with bad information. Anne, John,
Wendy, Philip, and the boys, then, needed to do
more than figure out whether and how to involve
Mr. Cantor in their advance planning conferences.
They also had to figure out what needed to be
decided in these conferences. And to do that, they
had to gather a fair amount of information. This is
not an easy task, because services for the aged and
for dementia sufferers are scattered; there's no central clearinghouse. So both children had to put in
long and sometimes frustrating sessions on the
telephone.

Anne, John, and their families had an even
harder job as well. They had to figure out how to
put together a fair and reasonable strategy for car-

ing in the light of the many different needs that confronted them. Like almost everybody else, they believe that fairness is as important a part of good moral decision making as is good information, but agreeing on what's fair in a particular case is often very difficult.

This was another job that couldn't be done without better information about what kinds of help their father was likely to need over time, and what kinds of help were actually available. Some of this information came from his doctor, some from the Alzheimer's Association, and some from books. Some also came from the planning conferences themselves, as each learned more about the others' situations, and looked for ways to fit new challenges as comfortably as possible into their established ways of living. They discovered that a fair amount of the information they needed was readily at hand, in themselves and their own lives, in what they valued, and in what mattered most to those they loved. Weighing all this information allowed them to get a better sense of what was possible if they were to help their father and still keep faith with their other responsibilities and commitments.

One effect of their early discussions was that John stopped insisting on having the money question settled his way. He could see that not everyone was willing to fall into line with his plan—that in fact, money was a very divisive topic. Rather than get bogged down in disagreement, he realized that it would be a good idea to see what financial issues they could agree on before they started on the controversies.

Anne consulted a lawyer to help with the financial part of her father's advance planning, and got a very careful explanation of what their legal options were. In the end, they decided that his money should be used mainly to provide for his care and comfort. Here's how they reasoned.

"It'll save trouble all the way around if Pop gives one of us power of attorney now," said Anne to John over the phone. "Otherwise, when he's really out of it and we have to pay bills or sell his house or whatever, we'll have to go to court and that's time-consuming, not to mention expensive. I think he'd be willing to let one of us *handle* his money, so long as he feels that nobody's trying to take it away from him."

"Of course nobody's trying to take it away from him. I was trying to shelter it so that nobody *could* take it away from him. I've been saying all along that he should be calling the shots here. It's his money. Absolutely. He has a perfect right to do anything he wants with it."

"Right. And our job is to try to figure out what that is, because he doesn't want to talk about it. You know, this would be a lot simpler if we could just lift up the top of his head and see what preferences he's carrying around in there. Because, as you say, we're only supposed to make sure that the money's used the way he'd prefer, without—"

"What?"

Anne was silent for a moment. "Well, I was going to say without considering anything or anybody else. But I wonder if I believe that. I mean, maybe it's not just Pop's preferences, but Pop himself—all of him—we're supposed to think about when we have to decide things for him."

"What do you mean?"

"Well, I was thinking about what we'd do if Pop's mind was just fine and he decided to spend all his money at the races or on a luxury cruise, even though he knew you needed it desperately and had never asked him for any kind of loan before. I think I'd argue with him. I'd tell him he'd always been too good a person to suddenly stop caring about the people who love him and need him. I'd tell him he couldn't do what he wanted just because he felt like it, and he ought to care about doing what's right."

"Okay. That's nice. So?"

"So, he'd agree with me. That's how he brought us up, for heaven's sake. So how come now that we have to make decisions for him, we're suddenly changing the rules and considering only what he might like for himself? Why aren't we also thinking about his commitments to things like justice and honesty, courage, compassion for people, kindness, how much he loves us? I guess I think if we're really looking after him right, we have to care about those things for him too."

John and Anne talked this idea over for a while and came to believe that, within limits, anyway, they did want to consider how their decisions on their dad's behalf fit within these broader moral commitments. Coming back to the question of how to manage their dad's money, they asked themselves whether anyone would be treated unfairly or unkindly or otherwise harmed if the money were spent to keep Pop comfortable. Was there anything nasty or selfish, if you stood in Pop's shoes, about spending the money this way?

They decided there wasn't. Pop and Mom had helped both kids when they were getting started in the world. By now, while neither child was exactly flush, both were certainly self-sufficient, and perfectly willing to acknowledge that they'd had more than their share of their father's generosity. Spending the money on him, now that he had special needs, seemed like a good and decent thing to do.

As for Mr. Cantor's medical needs, John and Anne discussed possible future care scenarios with his physician and with a geriatric nurse-practitioner they knew. Both were extremely helpful—particularly their nurse friend, who was able to tell them what might happen through stories drawn from her own experience.

Not everyone, of course, is in a position to enjoy this kind of consultation. But some people don't recognize the resources they do have. Although busy health care professionals don't always initiate the necessary conversations with family members, they will often respond generously if someone in the family gets a discussion going. In addition, advice about nonmedical matters can sometimes be had from local Alzheimer's support groups and the local Agency on Aging. And there are plenty of written sources of information on specific practical issues such as keeping the person physically oriented and making the house safe, or that survey the entire range of problems. Some of these sources are listed at the back of this book.

FURTHER DOWN THE ROAD

During this process of putting together contingency plans, Anne's distrust of John decreased. She came to believe that he was really interested in doing the right thing, that he wouldn't weasel out of helping and wouldn't try to grab what he could for himself. They still had some disagreements, but Anne felt much safer than before, because she now believed there was no hidden agenda lurking beneath their arguments.

John, for his part, got a much better sense of Anne's needs. He started taking her fears about his sexism seriously. From the start, if you had asked him, "Should female relatives have to do more of the caring, just because they are female?" he would have answered, "Certainly not." But he did not yet see that, if he weren't careful, he might try to foist off extra chores on Anne—without realizing that he was falling into the very pattern he had consciously rejected. Seeing things from her point of view, however, soon made it clear to him how much Anne had at stake, and this gave him a more vivid idea of what shouldering his own fair share might mean.

The most important thing that happened was that, in spite of Mr. Cantor's unwillingness to talk about his future, his kids eventually got a better sense of what kind of care he would be comfortable with. This knowledge was going to be helpful when decisions had to be made down the road.

Mr. Cantor had told John emphatically that he didn't ever want to be hooked up to a machine that did his breathing for him. And everybody agreed they would never let this happen. But as their doctor explained to them, they were thinking about the matter too simply. Respirator-assisted breathing might be all wrong for Mr. Cantor if it merely made his dying a longer, more drawn-out business. It might be just *right* for him, though, if he were suddenly in a crisis situation where he needed a boost; in that case he might soon be able to breathe again on his own.

Actually, the doctor added, even this rule of thumb wasn't all that helpful. While you might want the respirator for an emergency tomorrow, after ten years with Alzheimer's, you might not want to bother any longer. The same is true for cardiopulmonary resuscitation (CPR). If Mr. Cantor's heart suddenly stopped beating tomorrow, CPR would be appropriate; in ten years, it definitely wouldn't be. But in between, there would be a considerable gray area. If John is supposed to make the call, to what should he look for guidance?

John and Anne, with their spouses and kids, resolved that they would look, not so much to rules or to procedures, but *to Pop:* the man they knew now and had always known, their father and grandfather, the man who was sometimes irritable but always decent and human. They thought they could find in the patterns of his earlier life, in his former likes and dislikes, in his personal style and moral convictions, the guidance they would need now that his care and his dignity were both in their keeping.

Is Advance Planning for Everyone?

Some people might feel that the Cantors' approach to the problem doesn't fit their own family very well. That may be because the family is already too burdened, or too spread out, or too dysfunctional to present any kind of united front against a dementing disease. But it may be because the Cantors' approach feels too formal, too idealized, too much like a business transaction. It may not feel enough like the way people in their own family relate to one another.

It's true that the Cantors' procedure is fairly formal. For Anne and John, it was useful to think of what they were doing as a special process, with special rules and procedures: Anne wrote down summaries of their discussions and got everyone, including her dad, to agree to what she had written. Such formality worked well for this family—as it might in your own—because the people within it didn't fully trust one another. The formality was a way of dealing with suspicion.

Anne was on her guard, concerned that old patterns in the relationship with her brother might reassert themselves, suspicious that her commitment to caring for her dad was greater than John's, fearful that she might be stuck with an unfair amount of work. The very fact that the decision making was given a special context made it easier for her to reconcile what she felt she owed her father, what she felt she owed other members of her family, and what she owed herself. John, too, found the approach comfortable; it reminded him a bit of the negotiations that sometimes went on at work, and because of that association he was more inclined to take the family conferences seriously.

But such an association, for many people, might be just the problem. For these people, caring for a loved one with dementia isn't just a job, and families aren't little corporations. "Negotiations" are what entrepreneurs do, not sisters and brothers, husbands and wives, parents and children. For people who feel this way, the special sense of solidarity and affection that can bind family members together and give them strength might seem undercut rather than strengthened by the "businesslike" atmosphere that worked for John and Anne.

Perhaps for some families, questions like "What shall we do when Dad is unable to bathe himself?" or "How do we decide when to take the car keys from Mom?" or "When should we stop life-sustaining medical treatment?" don't really arise. The traditions of these families are strong and clear enough so that these questions and others like them are already answered—or at least the *way* in which they'll be answered is clear.

For most families, however, we think the answers to these questions are not so clear. While their members are held together by ties of affection and obligation, there will still be conflicts, largely because these ties are so numerous and so important. It isn't simply parents or spouses that matter in our family lives. Our children matter, and our siblings matter, and we matter, and the decisions we make need to respect all those different connections.

Advance planning sessions within families shouldn't operate by the rules of the market, where you try to cut the best deal you can for yourself while the other guys look out for themselves. But if we are to succeed in gathering the family's strength, making the best possible decisions, and fairly apportioning the burdens, something like a deliberate and self-conscious process of sorting things out and coming to agreement is going to have to occur. There are good reasons to talk things over. As the Cantors discovered, where there's some kind of solidarity to build on, talking can not only restore trust, it can also help people who've known each other for years to come to a new understanding of who they are together.

3

A Semblance of Normality

MARIE PYNE hates to be dependent on her husband Roy. *He* depends on *her*—always has—and that relationship isn't supposed to be turned upside-down. Besides, Marie really never has trusted him very much outside his own line of work. He was pretty good at operating earth-moving machinery, but that was about as far as it went. As for housekeeping or, years ago, taking care of the kids when they were sick, forget it.

He's got to take care of Marie now, though. She's been told that she has "dementia of the Alzheimer type," but she hasn't been able to take that fact in. Still, her dementia has progressed to the point where considerations of safety require Roy to keep a close eye on her. She's been burning herself regularly when she tries to cook dinner, and she finds that driving her car—even in daylight, even in her own neighborhood—is like entering a labyrinth.

Giving up the kitchen was a real hardship for Marie. She had been trying desperately to hang on, restricting her menu to simple meals, but the struggle was frustrating and painful. When Roy took away the microwave because she kept putting metal containers in it, she accused him of breaking it and hiding the pieces. She had always blamed him for being clumsy and stupid, so now, even though he knows she isn't responsible for what she says, her accusations hit home, hurting him the same way they always had. When he started unplugging the stove at night so she wouldn't burn herself while he was sleeping, he was careful to "fix" it in the morning with her watching—as if to prove to her that he wasn't clumsy and stupid after all.

For Marie, the idea of giving up driving was even more traumatic than curtailing her cooking, because of the loss of control and independence it represented. When Roy became convinced that she was starting to be a genuine hazard to herself and to other people, he tried to talk to her about it, but this made her frightened and defensive. It was no wonder, Roy thought. She was fighting to hang on to something crucial—her sense of herself as the person she'd always been. She wouldn't—couldn't—listen to Roy's pleading. For his part, he didn't like the idea of taking the car keys away from her by force. So for quite a while Roy simply made it his business to ride in the car with her any time she drove.

Roy was every bit as unwilling as Marie to see himself thrust into a caretaking role at his time of life. If anything, he tended to deny Marie's progressive loss of abilities longer than she did. The idea of his being "in charge" seemed as inappropriate and unlikely to him as it did to her.

The Pynes' career-oriented children, who live in distant cities, seem a little remote from their parents. There never was any one sharp break, no incident to which a person could point and say, "That's why their kids are so alienated." The fact remains, however, that Marie and Roy have been dealing with Marie's dementia on their own, except for Roy's niece Kathy, who stops by once or twice a week.

Marie's dementia is no longer merely a vague threat sending out ominous signals, but a daily reality, making everything about her life harder and more frightening than ever before. This is a time when Roy and Marie face difficult problems: for example, how to understand the shift in who is depending on whom, and how to balance risks to Marie—and to others—against the importance of helping her retain some degree of independence. The Pynes also face the challenge of defining what it means to live honestly together in the face of dementia. And as if all that weren't enough, Roy is taking on another new role: keeping faith with Marie's old self while he tries to understand and respond to her new reality.

Doing all this with grace will require a certain kind of thoughtful and imaginative caregiving, and Roy hasn't yet shown a great deal of enterprise in that direction. He could hardly be expected to, when he's got both hands full just struggling with the fact of his wife's illness. It's hard to summon up the sort of hope that spurs you to insight and creativity when you are facing a disease whose unavoidable conclusion is so profoundly depressing.

Despite his unpromising track record, however, Roy is slowly managing to come around. He is learning not merely to cope, but to do so with a kind of flair that surprises him as much as anyone. While still a reluctant cook and an indifferent housekeeper, he has come to an insight. He understands Marie's need to maintain what she can of the life she has always led, and, in small but important ways, he's being creative about how to help her do this.

Putting on fresh lipstick just before leaving the house was always part of Marie's daily routine— she didn't feel completely dressed without it. This had sometimes amused Roy, and sometimes (when it looked as if they would be late) slightly annoyed him. But most of the time he didn't think of it at all, until he started to notice that she couldn't get her lipstick on straight anymore.

One day she burst into tears as she struggled to do it. "My mouth is too little," she wailed. "I can't seem to aim at it today." Roy tried to help her, but the tube felt awkward in his hand and he had no idea how you put the stuff on, anyway. His incompetence only made things worse. Marie was too irritable to hold still for long. He felt he really *was* being clumsy and stupid, while she took his fumblings as fresh evidence of the fact that if she didn't do something herself, it wouldn't be done properly.

"I'm sorry, hon," Roy said after a few days of the lipstick wars. "I can't seem to get the hang of it. Does it really matter so much? You look fine without lipstick. Why don't you just stop wearing it?"

Marie couldn't stand this. Everything was being taken away from her, no matter how hard she tried just to be normal. Well, the world might be crumbling around her, but a lady never left the house without lipstick, and she wasn't about to start now. She could apply it herself if she had to. And she did. Badly.

Roy could have left the matter there, but the truth of it was that he was embarrassed by how she looked. He wasn't proud of this; he tried not to let it bother him; but she'd always been neat and tidy in her appearance, and now—! Besides, if he let her go out in public like that, people would start treating her differently, and that was the last thing she needed. So he'd have to come up with a second strategy. He'd just have to learn to use lipstick better.

He went into the bathroom, shut the door firmly, and practiced on his own lips until he got the hang of it. Brother, he thought, looking at himself in the mirror. Wouldn't the guys on the crew pay money to look at me now. All I need's a blond wig and falsies and I'm Marilyn Monroe. He grinned, washed off his mouth, and tried again. Having followed this up with a little extra experimentation on Marie, he can now apply lipstick for her with tolerable accuracy.

Something interesting happened as Roy learned a little cosmetology. Marie's daily routine became a shared ritual. She's grateful to him for helping her in this important way, and has begun to think he's not so clumsy after all. He's kind of handy, really. She supposes he could do some of the household chores she's tired of doing. And she likes having him put her lipstick on—it's kind of sexy, in a way.

Soon Roy got creative about other things as well. Marie had always been the "money person" in their house. Over the years, Roy brought home most of it, but it was always Marie who paid the bills, balanced the checkbook, and took care of the taxes. She struggled gamely on with these tasks too—longer than she should have, given the resulting confusions in their bank account. For a while, it looked as if the checkbook were going to have to go the way of the microwave. But now Roy has made it possible for her to feel that she is continuing to handle money, even though she is no longer up to it. He made a list of all the shops she was likely to patronize—her hairdresser, the grocer, the pharmacy. He made the rounds, explained the situation, and suggested a way Marie could continue to do business with them. Marie now pays for her purchases with checks that have been stamped "void." Her bills are actually sent to Roy every month, and he covers them out of his own account. He was concerned that the "void" stamp would give away the game, but Marie never seems to notice. It didn't occur to him that, although he was trying to be kind, these business people might start to treat Marie the way he'd feared they would if he let her go out of the house with her lipstick on crooked. That's just what the hairdresser did.

Sometimes Roy's bag of tricks is empty. Marie has occasional bouts of what would in a healthy person be considered bizarre nastiness. During a trip to the grocery store, for example, she suddenly began to shout at Roy. She yelled at him to go away and stop bothering her, telling the other customers that he was trying to steal her food. Roy was so distressed he couldn't even move, and simply stood there staring at her. Then she wrenched the cart away and started to slam it repeatedly into his shins. Mercifully, a neighbor who happened to be getting her groceries at the same time, was able to distract Marie. She soon forgot all about the frightening man who had tried to take her cart, and went home peaceably with her husband. This left Roy not only sore of shin, but extremely sore of heart. Marie's outburst angered and depressed him. It also scared him. His sense of who he was in relation to Marie had been a good part of what kept him going. His belief that he was doing a really good job of caring for her, much better than anyone could have anticipated, had been another source of strength. Now both of these beliefs were called into question. How could he continue to do a good job when she was nasty and abusive, and didn't even recognize him? Who *was* he in relation to this strange and ugly person? He hadn't realized her dementia was so advanced.

CHANGES

The ways in which Marie's and Roy's roles have shifted are painful, bewildering, and upsetting. The roles that make up our lives—particularly those we have lived with for years, and which absorb our time, energy, and creativity—become the pegs on which we hang our identities as the particular persons we are. When a dementing disease strikes, those basic roles change for both patient and caregiver, and identities can come unstuck.

Roy and Marie have to accept the fact that some changes are inevitable, and that all the kindness, empathy, and creativity in the world can't reverse the degeneration in Marie's brain. Some of her losses create problems the couple can't solve, problems that won't go away even if they can come up with the right strategies, get access to the right resources, enlist the support of friends and family. They are problems that Roy and Marie somehow must learn to live with.

For Roy, the main task became accepting what can't be changed with as little resentment as possible. This is never easy, and it has to be done day by day. As he struggled to live with what he couldn't fix, it struck Roy that maybe what he needed to do was to examine his ideas about what a human life is supposed to be like. Maybe he needed to change some of them.

This occurred to Roy when he visited a day care center shortly after Marie was diagnosed. Thinking that sometime in the future they might need such a program, he visited one that offered "stimulating and structured activities" to people with dementia while their family members enjoyed a little time off from caregiving. Through a window, he watched a group of women standing up and singing "You Are My Sunshine" while swaying back and forth to the music. The women were smiling and animated. In fact, to all appearances they were having a great time.

It was their very enjoyment that got to Roy. The idea that a person's life might come to *this,* that a person would be challenged and entertained by what looked like a kindergarten exercise, seemed to him disgusting and absurd. The idea that his own Marie was probably headed in that direction was bitter beyond words. At the same time, Roy also could see in these women a frightening image of himself in his own future, swaying back and forth and crooning half-remembered words to childish tunes.

However, as Roy watched one white-haired woman turn gracefully as she sang, something changed inside him. Suddenly, he simply couldn't see that woman, Marie, or himself as people who had completely lost their dignity. Perhaps, although it was sad, there was nothing especially awful about a dementing disease—not in the sense that it could really destroy a person's dignity. Dementia produces plenty of undesirable changes, Roy thought, but maybe not the loss of dignity. Maybe that's produced not so much by the disease as by having the wrong idea of what it is to be human. Maybe the lives of these smiling, singing, swaying women had frightened him because there was something the matter with his idea of what life was supposed to be. Many of us tend to blend our mental images of "dignified person" with our images of "productive, highly competent person," forgetting, perhaps, that none of us start out that way. We won't all end up competent, either. Maybe, Roy thought, the loss of competency isn't a cause for deep humiliation, but a part of the human story that may befall any of us. It's one way of experiencing the decline toward death. As such, it's a part of the poignancy and mystery of human life, not something outside humanity, not something completely foreign to us.

The change in Roy's outlook has done a lot to help him live day to day as Marie's disease worsens. Although he wasn't able to communicate his insight to Marie in words, the good effect it had on his own emotions did end up being communicated to her; the more calm and collected he could be, the less anxious and agitated she was. Roy had made a positive adjustment to change in his life.

While some changes have to be accepted through such adjustments in our images and ideals, others can be resisted, met more actively, influenced for better or worse. A major challenge in taking care of demented people is telling the difference between the two kinds of change. As we've observed before, family members can "cooperate" with dementia by treating an ill loved one in ways that speed up the loss of ability and self-concept. Or they can resist this process, finding new resources for extending abilities and improving attitudes. People's relationships, their very identities, are at stake in our responses to dementia. Making the distinction between what changes can be resisted or redirected, and what changes cannot, is a crucial part of the family caretaker's task.

She Might Get Hurt

Kathy came over to have a cup of coffee with her uncle Roy one day when Marie was at the day care center. She had an agenda. When was he going to take the car keys away from Aunt Marie?

"I'm terrified when I think of her on the road, even with you along. She'll kill you both one of these days." Kathy opened the drawer in the end table next to the couch, pulled out a coaster, and set her mug down on it. "It's over two years since she got lost driving home from my house that time. Don't you remember how frantic we were? I simply can*not* understand why you'd let her keep taking such risks."

"I know, I know. I worry about it all the time," Roy said. "But try to look at it from Marie's point of view. Think what it means to her."

"It means a car wreck waiting to happen," Kathy sniffed.

"It means she's normal," Roy contradicted, emphatically stirring a spoonful of sugar into his coffee. "It means she's an independent adult who can go places on her own and do things for herself like anybody else. If she can still get to the grocery store, she feels useful. She feels like she's still keeping house for me."

"Yes, but it's all playacting. She's *not* normal.

It's time to face facts, Uncle—she's not up to driving anymore."

"She's already lost so much, Kath," Roy pleaded. "She had to quit work, she doesn't see her friends much anymore, she doesn't get the pleasure out of cooking that she used to. If I take the car away from her, what's she got left? It's such a comfort to her that she can still drive. It makes her feel like things aren't so bad after all."

Kathy kicked off one shoe and drew her leg up under her, as if she were settling in for a long debate. "You're only thinking about Aunt Marie though, aren't you? What about all those other people who could lose their lives when she gets behind the wheel? It's sheer luck that she hasn't run over a little kid or had a head-on collision with somebody by now."

"Yeah, but everybody takes risks. They let fifteen-year-olds drive, even though most of 'em haven't got the sense God gave a canary. Taking chances doesn't have anything special to do with Marie being sick—*everybody* takes chances of one kind or another, every day, because that's the only way to get what you want. We live with risks all the time. The car companies have the know-how to make cars safer than they make 'em, but doing it would jack up the price, so we settle for 'safe enough.' And we know we could save lives if we lowered the speed limit, but we don't. We let people take chances."

"Within limits! We don't let babies play on the highway. At least most of us don't." Kathy reached for her mug and shot a withering glance at her uncle.

"Marie's not a baby," Roy said quietly. "She's a grown woman with a lot of dignity and she needs me to help her stay as strong and independent as she can. I'm trying to keep her from hurting anybody, and I think if I'm in the car I can do that. She's been so scared of losing her way that she doesn't mind having me ride with her so long as she can drive. If that changes—if it gets to where I can't count on her not to go off by herself—then I'll take her keys. But it'll hurt her."

The question of driving involved risk to other people. This was different from the question of cooking. Because Roy had done what he could to reduce the chances of fire in the kitchen, the only person Marie endangered there was herself. By not interfering with her when she continued to take that risk—apart from letting her know of his newly developed fondness for cold meals—Roy honored Marie's fullness as a person. Even more than the cooking itself, Marie valued her role as the one who fed her family. And there was another important part of her identity at stake here: she had never been the kind to be discouraged from doing something simply because there was discomfort or even danger involved.

So, although he really couldn't consult with

Marie about her "informed preference" concerning the danger versus the benefits of continuing to cook, Roy was guided by his memory of Marie's past, as well as his awareness of the continuing stake she had in maintaining her identity as the person who provided her family with meals.

As for her driving, although Marie continued to do it for quite a while after her dementia started to make itself felt behind the wheel, she limited herself more and more as time went on. Her biggest problem was always losing her way, rather than erratic or dangerous driving as such. With Roy in the car, the direction problem was solved, and avoiding driving in town, at night, or during bad weather lessened other dangers.

LIVING HONESTLY

It isn't enough to know when to continue risky activities and when to stop them. A loving caregiver will also be interested in cushioning the loss for the person who is ill with a dementing disease. Are there ways of helping that person hang on to the sense of importance and competence associated with activities that are no longer appropriate?

This was a question that interested Roy. It's why he made his special arrangement with the local merchants. While Marie couldn't be trusted to do the family books any longer, or to use a checkbook properly, she could be given the semblance of these responsibilities. Not only did Roy give her the checks stamped "void," he also got her a calculator with extra large keys and an especially bright display, to give Marie the sense that, despite her losses, she could still handle the finances. In fact, Roy took the whole thing over himself; the calculator was just a prop in the performance.

So Marie got to keep, longer than she otherwise would have, some things quite precious to her: a sense of usefulness and a feeling of continuity in a world that was changing with terrifying speed. Or at least she got to hang on to the *belief* that she had these things, and she was no longer in much of a position to distinguish what she believed from what was, in fact, the case. But without knowing it, Marie may have lost something else she had always prized: the kind of honesty that had consistently been a part of her relationship with Roy. In exchange for receiving the *impression* that she had kept her adult status, she may have lost the *reality* of being treated with the dignity and respect to which an adult is entitled.

There is, of course, another way of interpreting what has occurred. Her husband is creatively seeking a new vocabulary with which to express something that is true about Marie, but which cannot any longer be said in the old ways. Marie is still a person of substance and worth, as her history and present status attest. However, because of the handicaps that come along with her damaged brain, the typical ways of acknowledging her status simply don't work. Seen from this perspective, Roy's creative accommodations are ways to express a "deeper truth" about Marie, and, therefore, are not false or deceptive in any important sense.

What's the correct way to understand what is going on here? Is Roy trading off illusion for reality? If so, is it a good trade? Or is he using unusual means to express something that, fundamentally, is true? Sometimes Roy thinks he's been extremely clever about the whole thing, and that thought gives him some sorely needed affirmation of his ability to cope. But other times his stratagems make him nervous. How should he feel? Proud? Uncomfortable? Both? Neither?

Truth-telling has to be more the rule than the exception if we are to relate effectively to others. If deception were the prevailing practice, no one could trust anyone and much of our daily lives would be paralyzed. The amount of deception that does exist in daily life brings with it tremendous social costs.

But it seems equally true that a little judicious molding of the truth can sometimes have good effects. What Roy did with the neighborhood merchants has on the whole been extremely good for Marie, and there seems to have been only a little negative fallout. How could this possibly be faulted?

To get a perspective on the question, try to remember how you felt the last time you found out that someone had lied to you—even if the lie was "for your own good." It is likely your first thought wasn't, "Were the consequences of this lie good overall?" More probably, you felt hurt, offended, yanked around, manipulated by the deceiver—despite all the good intentions, and even despite good results.

This kind of response suggests that truth-telling has a dimension that reaches beyond immediate results, to the question of respect. Many people feel that to be the subject of deception—again, even in their own interests—is not to be treated with full respect. And when the person doing the deceiving is someone they have special reason to trust, they may feel that the covenant between them—the implicit promise to keep faith with each other—has been broken. Deceiving people is not wrong simply because it makes them feel bad: they feel bad because they were wronged. And anyway, it would be wrong even if they *didn't* feel bad.

Marie, most probably, won't feel bad. She is not going to see through any of Roy's deceptive strategies. But that doesn't mean he is honoring her dignity or treating her with the respect that is her due—especially considering that her dignity is already in a perilous condition.

For his part, Roy might reply that truth-telling is no longer the way to show respect for Marie, that being honest is made much more difficult because of her dementia, and that we ought to cut him a lot of slack as he tries hard to come up with ways of making life easier for someone he loves. It's not right to tell a lie so you can put somebody at an unfair disadvantage, but that's very different from deceiving a loved one in an effort to be kind.

If Roy said this he'd be right. But even lying out of love can be an ethically dangerous strategy. For one thing, there's something seductive about feeling that you are entitled to take liberties with the truth. Lying to or deceiving others is a way of gaining power over them, and that is surely an attractive idea to many of us much of the time. It can be difficult to guard against this seduction, especially if we feel forced to give in to it in one particular area of our lives, as someone might who was caring for a demented spouse.

Further, many people would, if pressed to think about it, feel some compunction about lying even to children (as opposed to playing with them in ways that blur fact and fantasy). Even assuming that the children wouldn't penetrate the deception and that some good end was in view, we might feel we shouldn't lie. These scruples suggest that lying raises moral problems even when the dupe is not a fully rational and competent person.

Roy might make one last protest here. It's not as if he deliberately set out to deceive Marie. She's got these delusions that she's still able to make financial transactions. He's simply going along with her because breaking down a demented person's delusions can be shattering.

Again, Roy is partly right. Breaking down a demented person's delusions can indeed be shattering, but going along with a delusion is rather different from helping to create one. When Roy rides with Marie in the car, he doesn't pretend he's not there so she can feel she's doing it on her own. When he gives her checks stamped "void," however, he's actively building on her delusional state.

Shading the truth—even outright lying—can achieve important goals for people in Roy's position. But it has its costs. It ought not to be seen as simply another routine strategy to be used, even with very kindly motives, when interacting with demented people. Insofar as possible, the presumption in favor of avoiding deceit ought to be seen as holding for demented as well as nondemented people.

CREATIVE COPING AND A SPECIAL KIND OF STRESS

We have seen Marie and Roy both making creative accommodations to their new situation, and finding some degree of success, of solace, even of renewed intimacy, in doing so. Routines have been ruptured, presenting Roy with a pointed invitation to think more seriously about his wife and what her life is like than he has done for a long time. As a partial consequence, he has been thinking somewhat less about himself.

This has been tremendously helpful to him as he has adjusted to his new life with Marie. The lipstick ritual is an excellent example of how creative coping has worked for them both. Roy has always said he'd do anything for Marie, but he never anticipated that "doing anything" might involve learning how to put on lipstick. However, thinking about Marie and her needs in a newly concentrated way brought him to it, and the result has been moments of closeness between them, moments they both cherish.

All these accomplishments—facing changes, managing risks, rethinking what it is to live honestly with each other, and creative coping—grew out of Marie and Roy's joint involvement in maintaining Marie's sense of self. What the two of them have to draw on for this task is the integrity of their relationship, their loyalty to each other, and Roy's loving imagination. Roy has become actively involved in maintaining his wife's sense of self, and therefore, we suggest, her actual personhood as well. Because people are, to some extent at least, formed and maintained by their interactions with others, they can also be eroded by the treatment they receive. If a person is thrust by others into the role of "senile old lady" it can become very difficult to resist this characterization and remain alive to other, equally valid characterizations. Marie may have dementia, but she is also a housewife, a mother, a neighbor, a friend. When she is in a fragile and confused state, she will require extra help from others to affirm these very important parts of herself that no one used to question.

There is, however, a special kind of stress lurking here, one that we will simply flag now, and explore in depth in later chapters. As Roy devotes more and more of his time, energy, and creativity to shoring up Marie's identity, what will happen to his own? Might it ever be the case that the demands and strains of caretaking become just so burdensome that he ought to refuse them?

Here, we aren't imagining conflicting duties to other people. Roy, fortunately, is pretty free of those. Rather, we are imagining conflicts *within Roy himself*. If a drastic change in her social context can help hold Marie together, in spite of her neurological disorder, might a drastic change in his social context pull Roy apart, in spite of his intact nervous system?

It's lucky in a way that Roy has not had the kinds of relationships and absorbing hobbies it would be painful to put on hold while Marie's care absorbs more and more of his time and attention. Nor is the task of caring for her so demanding that he literally has no time for himself. The Alzheimer day care program gives him some chance to recharge his own batteries. As we will see, however, not everyone is so well positioned, nor remains so all the way through the course of the disease.

4

From Home
to Nursing Home

ELAINE GIBBARD was diagnosed as having Alzheimer's disease five years ago. Her husband died the year before last, and about six months ago she moved into her son Alan's home. Alan lives in a small Cape Cod house with his wife Marjorie and their two daughters, Beth and Judy. Marjorie is an RN who works part time at the local hospital; Alan is an insurance adjuster; the kids are in high school.

Grandma Gibbard's arrival had a dramatic impact right from the start. For one thing, everybody lost their bedroom. The girls had to move in together, and as it made sense to put the two single beds into the master bedroom, Alan and Marjorie's double bed went into much smaller quarters. More pressure was put on the Gibbards' only—and already heavily trafficked—bathroom. Marjorie started to turn down extra shifts at work. Even the usual three a week became too much for her, and she could no longer be at the hospital when Alan was on the road.

To a large extent, these changes were anticipated and the family had done its best to prepare for them. Alan, Marjorie, Beth, and Judy had had a rather intense series of discussions just after Alan's father's death. At that point, Alan was pretty hesitant about asking Grandma to live with them, but there didn't seem to be any other choice. His sister and her husband had their hands full already with a chronically ill child and with layoffs at work, and it was clear that Grandma couldn't live on her own much longer. So Alan and Marjorie and the girls tried hard to anticipate just what would be involved in taking care of her, and to get their feelings squarely behind what they all saw as their duty.

But despite this careful preparation, having Grandma in their home wasn't at all what they had thought it would be. Whether it was the doubly disorienting blows of her husband's death and her change of residence, or whether her dementia had just progressed farther than anyone realized, Grandma brought with her some problems that caught the family off guard. Uninterrupted sleep has become a luxury at the Gibbards'. Grandma often gets up in the middle of the night and wanders through the house, getting panicky and crying uncontrollably until someone—almost always

Marjorie, unless she is at work—gets up and puts her back to bed. Dinner is no longer a welcome pause in the day's occupation, when people can relax, spend some time together, and catch up on each other's lives. Grandma needs too much help with eating. She can't get dressed by herself either, but that's not so bad; Marjorie lays out two outfits and, when Grandma has chosen one, helps her into her clothes. They used to have a dreadful time getting Grandma to brush her teeth, but now, instead of telling her to do it and thereby inviting refusal, Marjorie asks her to choose between the red and the blue toothbrush, and Grandma brushes more willingly. Harder to deal with is Grandma Gibbard's occasional incontinence. She can't always control her bladder. And what is worse is that sometimes she doesn't recognize her daughter-in-law, or even her son; the girls seem like strangers to her much of the time. This frightens her, and when she is frightened, she is often loud and aggressive.

Family life isn't totally grim, though. One day Alan came across his mother chatting happily with the lady in a hoopskirt who forms part of the wallpaper pattern in the upstairs hall. His first thought was to try to call her back to a better sense of her surroundings, but then it struck him that she seemed to be having a nice little talk and there was no reason to interrupt. And the other night, Grandma announced to the family that she was going out dancing. The reality, of course, is that Grandma isn't going dancing. Her dementia has progressed to the point where she can't even be left alone. And this in turn has had serious consequences for the Gibbards' social life.

Since she moved into her son's home, Grandma never sees any of her old friends, and it's not certain she would recognize them if they did make the trip to her new neighborhood. Alan and Marjorie never go out as a couple any more, and having people in for an evening has become difficult and rare. Even the family circle is sorely reduced after dinner. Beth and Judy vanish between dinner and bedtime, and are seldom to be found around the house during weekends or school breaks. Marjorie and Alan have only the vaguest impression of what their daughters' friends are like, since neither Beth nor Judy ever invites them over.

As the Disease Progresses

By this point in the Gibbards' lives, the answers to many questions—about sharing tasks, about balancing care for Grandma against care for other family members, about the kind of medical treatment that will be most appropriate down the road—have already been worked out. The Gibbards did a fair amount of advance planning and preparation, a fair amount of negotiating about who does what. However, even though thought and care were expended on these questions, the questions themselves have now shifted in both foreseen and unforeseen directions, so that the old answers are no longer workable. That means the questions have to be raised again and the responses reconsidered.

There is no possibility at this point of Grandma's being directly involved in such discussions, of course. But if, several years ago when she could still be included, Marjorie and Alan had anticipated the need to rethink old plans and to make new ones, they might have asked her how she'd want them to go about reconsidering things as time went on. Her answers then might make her family feel more comfortable with the decisions they must still make now.

Suppose, for example, there had been earlier discussions about where Grandma would want to live as the disease progressed, and she had chosen to live with Alan and his family. Suppose further that, during the discussion, someone had brought up the possibility that the family's caring resources could give out, and that a nursing home might at some point become necessary. If Mrs. Gibbard had explicitly acknowledged this possibility, then an eventual move of that kind might be easier on everybody.

The Gibbards' discussions took place too late for that. In any case, the family had focused more on the impact of her moving *into* the house, and less on the impact of her leaving it again. Clearly, the Gibbards have a lot more to talk about as the ongoing reality of Grandma's extended, day-to-day care becomes more and more a part of everyone's life.

But what they face is not merely a matter of coming up with new plans of action in response to steadily changing needs. It's also a matter of accepting something that can't be changed. The Gibbards, already stressed by the illness, now have to cope with two simultaneous trends, each of which is heartbreaking and which together are tragic. While Mrs. Gibbard's need for care continually expands, her ability to participate meaningfully in family life keeps contracting. She is moving toward a time when, like a newborn, virtually all of her needs will have to be met by others. Unlike a newborn, however, she won't possess the vital sense of future promise, of new abilities flowering daily, that almost all babies have. And there is nothing her family can do about this.

The Gibbards, then, are faced with a huge challenge. How can they protect what they value about their life with Grandma when she is passing beyond the point of being able to recognize and interact with them? How can they come to terms with what is happening to this person they love? And how can they make the hardest decision they've ever faced as a family—entrusting

Grandma to a nursing home? In this chapter, we will focus on all these problems.

"WEAR AND TEAR" VS. "ADAPTATION"

"What I'm worried about," remarked Marjorie to Alan late one afternoon as Grandma dozed in front of the TV, "is that if we keep this up much longer we're going to wear ourselves right out. Keeping your mom from wandering off is getting to be a full-time job and we're all heading toward exhaustion. And look at how tense things are between us and the kids. I've been having one cold after another all winter, which is nothing but stress. You've been getting headaches. And Judy flunked math last term. At some point, the wear and tear on the family is going to be so enormous that we won't be able to keep Grandma at home anymore, and what'll we do then?"

Alan took two beers out of the refrigerator and reached for the bottle opener. "What'll we do?" he repeated. "We'll adapt. We'll grow. We'll learn how to cope with the challenges as they get more challenging." He poured beer into a glass and watched it foam up. "See, I think you've got the wrong idea about what people can stand. It's not like they only have X amount of care and compassion in them, and if somebody drains it all out before they fill it back up again, they're empty.

That's more like a gas tank than a person. Or like this beer glass. What're you, a beer glass?"

Marjorie took the glass and drank from it. "Better that than a gas tank, I guess. Remind me again why I'm not a beer glass?"

"Because you can expand your caring capacity. You can cultivate your resources until you've got more than you ever thought you could have. I've seen you do it. You're wonderful, Marge. You started out very loving, but dammit if you haven't grown about six sizes this last year. You aren't going to wear out or drain out. You'll just adapt."

"Yeah, well, maybe I do adapt. But I've been doing more than my share and I'm tired. How about you getting off your duff and growing a couple more sizes too? You can start by getting Grandma back to bed tonight."

Obviously, Marjorie didn't share Alan's rosy view, but as they kept talking, she came to think that maybe they both were right. Maybe she and Alan could keep up the home-based caregiving for the period of time when it was most important to Alan's mom. Maybe for just that long the family could keep adapting enough to shoulder the task. And maybe after a while, when that task became so heavy it really would wear them all out, when Grandma's care started to destroy other important parts of their lives, maybe then it would seem natural and appropriate to let the brunt of the care pass on to professionals. She'd feel awfully guilty about it, though.

Anyway, as Alan pointed out, they all *had* adapted. They had all been changed by the caregiving they'd been doing. Changes in routine had themselves become routine. What at first seemed like extraordinary problems become decidedly ordinary. But the idea wasn't just that people can get used to anything. Rather, Alan was arguing that providing care for his mom had transformed the caregivers. In his opinion, the experience of giving basic and intense care itself deepens and widens what the caregiver can do, and even who the caregiver is.

What happened, of course, is that the Gibbards both adapted *and* experienced wear and tear. The many tasks of caregiving became progressively less distressing but also more difficult. After a time, like other loving, well-motivated, and conscientious caregivers, they did simply become exhausted. Their own health got worse and their ability to honor other commitments was strained. Now the problem is figuring out how they can reduce wear and tear while increasing their ability to adapt, so that they can at least survive sharing their home with Grandma. Because they're still concerned about responding well to her great need, this is a moral question as well as a practical one.

WHERE THE RESOURCES CAN BE FOUND

One essential part of the Gibbards' strategy must be to get help from their community. They need to learn about sources of support, both practical and psychological. There may be ways to get temporary help that would allow Alan and Marjorie to get out together now and then. Perhaps there are affordable senior day care facilities that Mrs. Gibbard would like and that would make it easier for the girls to have their friends over. They can get information about these sources of help by phoning their local Agency on Aging or the Alzheimer's Association.

There may also be resources the family can tap into at home. Mrs. Gibbard's new environment may become less disorienting as she becomes more familiar with it, or even as she loses the ability to note the difference between the familiar and the strange. If letting a little time pass doesn't ease her disorientation, there may be changes and adjustments that her family can make in the home. Lights can be left on in hallways at night. The CD player can still play grunge rock bands, but also Grandma's old favorite—Mario Lanza singing songs from *The Student Prince*. And Mrs. Gibbard can be included in the daily chores that are familiar to her: whoever is putting dinner together or washing up afterward can take her into the kitchen, too.

Finally, there are resources in Alan, Marjorie, Beth, and Judy themselves, ways of thinking and feeling that may help to nurture their own caregiving inclinations and abilities. New ways of thinking about a situation are resources that can make it easier to respond (as Roy found out in the last chapter) without feeling defeated or devastated. And other inner resources can make it possible to stay better connected—both to the person who so often doesn't act or look like her old self anymore, and to one's own self, as well.

Staying Connected

Marjorie first figured out how to do what she calls staying connected to herself one day twenty years ago, shortly after she saw that she would have to give up the baby she was carrying for adoption. She hadn't meant to get pregnant—she was still in school, struggling to keep up her grades, with no prospects for her life unless she got her degree. Her boyfriend wanted to help, but he was as much of a kid as she and no better equipped for fatherhood than her sixteen-year-old brother. Her parents wouldn't take her in; she had nowhere else to turn. But how could she leave her own wonderful baby with strangers? It would tear her apart.

It was while she was numbly walking to class

one day in the middle of all this that she realized she could relate to herself as a deeply concerned, benevolent friend—a friend who loved her very much. From that viewpoint, she could feel enormous compassion for this young woman plodding along the sidewalk, wishing her well as she journeyed one year, five years, ten years down the road. It didn't take away the numbness in her legs or the pain in her heart, but it did seem to put it all into a richer context, one that made it easier for her to get unstuck, to start moving again with some sense that she wasn't completely alone, and that her life was very much worth living.

She has never gotten over the pain of having to give her baby up for adoption, but ever since, this memory of good friendship has been useful to Marjorie when she goes through difficult times. However hard her life may be, she always retains the sense that she is connected and not alone. And this sense, in its turn, helps her get through her troubles with more grace and less damage, less wear and tear, than she otherwise might experience.

When Marjorie was walking to class that day, it seemed to her that she had found a way of looking at her life that was both intimate and deeply engaged. She knew just what was going on, and she wasn't distorting how she felt about it. These weren't feelings of heroic self-denial, nor feelings that her problems were trivial compared to what others were going through, nor feelings of loyalty to the eternal verities, nor anything of that sort. She was buoyed up by her friendship for herself, but in a way that wasn't totally self-absorbed or dominated by the problem she faced at that moment in time. Rather, she allowed her loving concern for her own life and what was happening within it to spill over her tragedy and fit it into a broader vision.

What Marjorie experienced then was not simply a refined sort of egotism. She also started to see those around her in a more connected way, and hence, more sympathetically. She now knows that releasing whatever inner resources she has available to help her is in large part a matter of embracing the people in her life—including her mother-in-law—richly and deeply. Alan and the children have long been aware of this strategy for connecting to herself like a friend when times are hard. Can they, like Marjorie, achieve a perspective from which to "connect" to their sometimes nasty and always upsetting Grandma?

All the Gibbards have tried to cultivate this kind of connection these past several months. Mrs. Gibbard's presence in their home has been disruptive, distressing, difficult, and damaging. Despite their best efforts, they are all rather less in touch with one another than they were at this time a year ago, and everyone is feeling a sort of pervasive sadness. But they do realize that they are a part of something deeply important: the closing chapter in the life of someone they all love. Somehow, business as usual is just not fitting at such a time. Right now, life for the Gibbards is hard and sad—and at the same time, an invitation to love.

Because they've tried hard to reconnect themselves to their situation, Beth and Judy don't find it as shameful and socially upsetting as they did at first. Judy started thinking about how she'd react if all this were happening to a close friend, and on the strength of her reaction she found the courage to invite a few of her more thoughtful and sensitive friends home. She hasn't regretted it, even though one of her friends found it too uncomfortable an experience to want to repeat. At first that made Judy mad, but then she had to laugh at herself, since feeling "uncomfortable" was precisely why she herself had been staying away from home so much. As a result of her experiment, Judy's been able to cut her friend some slack—and cut herself some, too.

The effort to stay connected also helps everyone maintain a more vivid sense of Mrs. Gibbard than they otherwise might have. Rather than simply focusing on the old woman here and now—a woman who is being obstreperous, or a lot of trouble, or who doesn't seem to know these people who are all breaking their backs to take care of her, they keep in mind that Grandma brought with her into the present moment a full history, one in which all their own lives are deeply engaged. The family has tried to nourish this way of thinking by ransacking old albums and "keepsake" boxes for pictures, cards, and other mementos of Grandma's life, and the life they have shared together. Old photos have been dusted off and put in new frames around the house.

Staying connected to Grandma and to each other has made a difference in the family's experience of caring for her, and for one another as well. It isn't magic, of course; their situation remains difficult, distressing, and even damaging. But the grace that is growing allows them to feel the importance of what they're doing. It may extend their career as her primary caregivers. And it may also ease their own transition to a different kind of caretaking role, when and if Mrs. Gibbard leaves to take up residence in a nursing home.

THE NURSING HOME

Many of us dislike the thought of nursing homes, not only because of the not-so-distant scandals that have been associated with them, but also because they make us feel we've failed. The popular image of these homes has a lot to do with their history, which traces back to the poorhouses of the nineteenth century. It was a disgrace to have to go to the poorhouse—a sign of thriftlessness and lack of moral fiber. Shame attached to families who were so improvident as to be forced to resort to such places for care. Yet poorhouses, grim and punitive though they were, increasingly became a dumping ground for the old and infirm.

At the beginning of the twentieth century, state mental hospitals seemed like a more humane alternative, at least for the care of the demented elderly. At the same time, medical hospitals came to specialize in short-term, acute care. Nursing homes, some sponsored by churches and some intended to turn a profit, began to provide long-term care—increasingly, the care of the old. At mid-century, when the deinstitutionalization movement prompted state mental hospitals to discharge many of their aged residents to communities that, as it turned out, could not care for them, nursing homes became even more specialized. They became places where elderly people suffering from dementing diseases could go.

In the 1950s and 1960s, just at the time when mental hospitals were releasing their elderly patients, scandal after scandal gave nursing homes an even worse name. There were widespread reports of substandard care and outright physical abuse. There were shady financial practices, ranging from kickbacks and fraud to theft of residents' assets. Strict governmental oversight in the last fifteen years has begun to correct these evils, but the truth is that many nursing homes are still rather bleak and depressing places. Residents sometimes injure other residents or take their things; daily life can be extremely tedious and boring in the absence of structured activities; the surroundings can be grim and utilitarian; staff can be unresponsive or disrespectful of the person who is ill; and in even the best of homes there is no getting away from the clamor, the lack of privacy, the totality of the institution. The stigma of the poorhouse remains attached to nursing homes, and families still tend to blame themselves for having to "abandon" a loved one to them.

As it stands now, only 5 percent of the elderly spend any length of time in nursing homes, although that number will increase as the baby boomers grow old. Moreover, family abandonment of the elderly is relatively rare in the United States, where heavy care, often past the point of burnout, is the *norm* for family relationships. Most families will not consent to nursing home placement until their own caregiving capacities are exhausted, even though this is hard on both the frail elderly person and her or his family. The avoidance of institutional care is understandable. Nursing homes still summon up images of neglect, abandonment, and poverty, even though there have been significant attempts at reform.

The Gibbards found the idea of a nursing home so distasteful that they initially ruled it out altogether. They'd been having a hard time sorting through negative stereotypes and false pride whenever the subject came up. Finally, though, they reconsidered. They came to realize that at some point they might not be able to meet all of Mrs. Gibbard's needs, and they toured a facility that looked as if it could meet them. But they weren't ready to decide anything yet.

WHEN THE TIME COMES

Then one Saturday night Alan came home to find the family in an uproar. That afternoon when Beth, who had been the only one home with Mrs. Gibbard, was in the shower getting ready for an evening out, the old lady had wandered outside and disappeared. She had now been missing for more than five hours, and everyone was frantic. Marjorie had called the police and the two hospitals in town, but no one had seen anyone answering to Mrs. Gibbard's description.

The police eventually brought her home. Despite the latches Alan installed high up on all the doors leading outside, which everyone tried hard to remember to secure, the same thing happened in the middle of the night two weeks later. This time it was Alan who found her—in her nightgown in the snow, two miles from the house. "I was trying to go home," she sobbed. "I can't find Daddy."

After he and Marjorie warmed her and got her to bed, it was Alan's turn to cry. "I'm doing a lousy job of taking care of her, Marge. She's miserable and homesick and I don't know what to do about it. And look at you—you're worn out. What she needs is somebody with her all the time, day and night. And we haven't got the money for that, because I don't have a good enough job. Goddammit, I feel like I'm letting everybody down!"

Marjorie knew he wasn't letting anybody down and tried to tell him so. She didn't feel as angry as he, but she could match him guilt for guilt. She felt she was doing everything wrong, that she was failing, that this lovely woman who had always been so good to her and who was now so needy and vulnerable deserved far better than she was getting. And she also knew that she and Alan were in treacherous, unspoken agreement that the time had come to find a nursing home.

Treachery was the operative emotion here. They felt they were betraying Mrs. Gibbard. Surely, they thought, we could be working at it a *little* harder than we are. Surely we aren't giving 100 percent. Surely we could buy her just a little more time with us if we were more patient and less lazy. These emotions were strongest in Alan, of course, since it was his mother, and because of that, Marjorie didn't feel she could take the initiative. She could only look on, guilty, as Alan struggled with his feelings.

It was Judy who broke the impasse. She and Alan were sharing a late night snack at the kitchen table, waiting for Marjorie to come home from work. "You think Grandma's going to have to go to a home, don't you?"

"She's not going to a home. I promised her we'd never do that, and we're not going to."

"Yeah, but it's not that simple, is it? So you're wondering how you're going to live with yourself."

Alan didn't say anything. Judy pushed her plate aside and propped her elbows on the table. "I've been thinking about it, Daddy. Listen. You know how when there's a divorce, little kids are afraid that if their parents can stop loving each other, they could stop loving *them?* It doesn't work like that, but that's what little kids think. They get mixed up about what counts as a divorce and what doesn't." She smiled at him sadly, her face glowing in the lamplight. "If you put Grandma in a nursing home, you aren't divorcing her. It's a big change in the family, but it's not a divorce. You don't stop loving her. It doesn't work like that. It's pretty easy to get mixed up about it, though."

That moment was an important one for Alan. It didn't put an end to his guilt or allay his anger, but it unstuck him so that he and Marjorie could get serious about finding a nursing home that would meet his mother's needs. They checked out the six that were close enough for frequent visits, thinking these would be crucial for everyone's peace of mind. What they didn't know then, but were soon to discover, is that frequent visits were also important for building rapport with the nursing home staff. Residents who had family to communicate, translate, and advocate for them generally got better and more individualized care than those who didn't. The reason is that families serve as historians of a kind. They can tell the staff who this person had been: "She's too quiet. That's not like her. Maybe she's depressed, or not feeling good, or something's bothering her." By their presence, families can also set the staff an example of loving and respectful care.

For these reasons, the home had to be close by. But it also had to feel okay. Marjorie and Alan crossed three off the list right away because they felt unfriendly or unkempt or just—funny. Of the other three, St. Anne's had a Dementia Special Care Unit, designed to maintain residents' functioning as long as possible, and then, when the disease was advanced, to promote people's comfort rather than treat them with inappropriate, aggressive medicine. The Gibbards thought this facility would be better for Mrs. Gibbard than the others, so they put her on the waiting list.

They dreaded telling her, and when they did, it was as bad as they feared. First she cried, and then she yelled, and then she insisted that they get out of her house. By the next day, though, she had forgotten, so they let it alone temporarily. They hired an elder lawyer to help them do the paperwork and sort out the financial side of things. He was expensive but worth it, because he knew what needed doing and they didn't. When it was all done, they waited.

When the call came, they packed up Mrs. Gibbard's things and once again tried to explain to her where they were going. She couldn't seem to understand until Beth said, playfully, that they were taking her to a college where she'd learn to improve her memory. Alan shot her a very black look, but Grandma was interested. "College?" she beamed. "You know, I always wanted to go to college. Let's get in the car!" Rattled, but amused all the same, Marjorie and Alan helped her in and drove her to St. Anne's.

Leaving her there was dreadful. Alan was wracked by guilt and Marjorie felt she could never look her mother-in-law in the face again. There were so many old and ill people about, and some of them were making noises. Grandma's roommate seemed nice enough, but she followed Marjorie around wherever she went, and Grandma looked little and bewildered. But she told her roommate proudly, "I'm in college now." And while Alan felt he shouldn't let her keep thinking that, he also needed desperately to make things easier for her, and couldn't bring himself to correct her belief.

IN THE NURSING HOME

The Gibbards visited Grandma regularly—twice a week for a while. Although Alan got off to a bad start with the regular staff by being critical and demanding, Marjorie could see that Grandma was losing out because of this, and persuaded him to save his criticisms for things that really mattered. "The aides are only human," she urged. "Like anybody else, they do their work much better if they're admired and appreciated. Connect with them—you know yourself it's not easy looking after old people." They brought pictures of a younger Grandma to give the nursing home workers some sense of the whole of her life. They tried hard to supplement the direct knowledge the staff had of her now with their own knowledge of her past.

They learned it was also good to visit on the weekends, when the auxiliary staff was on duty. One Saturday when Alan arrived he found his mother wearing a diaper, due to a weekender's mistake. "Mom!" he exclaimed. "You don't need a diaper. Why didn't you tell the aide?"

"Oh, I thought they were trying something new."

For a time, Mrs. Gibbard actually seemed to do a little better than she had at home—partly because of the special programs in the dementia unit and partly, perhaps, because she was no longer in the sole care of exhausted and burned-out relatives. But after a year or so the days on which she was withdrawn, critical, and angry began to outnumber the "good" days, and visiting her came to be a real chore.

Marjorie and Alan were faithful about it, though. They were now visiting only once a week, but it *was* once a week, and Judy and Beth came once or twice a month. Conversations with Grandma were—well, weird—because she would say disconnected and cryptic things and you never knew who you were to her. Sometimes Beth was Mrs. Gibbard's daughter, sometimes her sister, sometimes her mom. And it was the same for Marjorie. It was easier if two or more of the family came together, because then they could at least talk to each other. It was also easier to visit together in Mrs. Gibbard's room than in the residents' lounge, because when she was in the lounge she felt the need to get up and look after the other visitors, bringing them magazines or the potted plants on the tables, or pulling up chairs for people to sit on.

Over time, the family got to know the other residents and some of their relatives, although not everyone had family to come and visit. Marjorie and Alan made a point of smiling and speaking to everyone, even though this sometimes invited more attention from a resident than they had bargained for. And almost every week Mrs. Rizzuto would come into Mrs. Gibbard's room when they were there and lie down on the roommate's bed. She couldn't speak much English, but Marjorie and Alan would nod and smile to her, and when the visit was over she would go back to her room. It seemed she needed visitors too.

As disconcerting, distressing, and upsetting as their visits could be, Alan and Marjorie continued to come. They could see it made a difference to the staff, not only because it was a way of keeping an eye on Mrs. Gibbard's care, but because faithful visiting demonstrated that they had a certain amount of "sweat equity" invested in Mrs. Gibbard's welfare. It gave them standing with the nursing home staff. They were listened to better than family members who came only a few times a year.

The Gibbards didn't visit simply as a means of maintaining good relations with Grandma's care-givers, however. Nor was it guilt alone that compelled them to come. These motives played their part, to be sure, but had they been magically removed, Marjorie and Alan, Beth and Judy would still have made their way to St. Anne's on a regular basis. It was a part of their covenant with Grandma. It was a way of keeping connected to her.

5

The Final Stages

RANDOLPH WOLTER, born in 1911, lost his father to the influenza epidemic that swept the country soon after Armistice Day. He weathered the Depression, which broke just as he was trying to get into the job market, and when war was declared after Pearl Harbor, he threw over his job at the garage and joined the Navy. He spent his war as a Seabee—a construction engineer—hopping from atoll to atoll in the Pacific Theater. His ship was nearly torpedoed once, he had a couple of minor construction accidents, and he came down with a nasty bout of malaria. None of that was particularly traumatic, but when enemy fire killed one of his buddies, a guy he'd grown particularly close to and who died in his arms, he couldn't seem to get over it. He talked of it often in later years—of how it frightened and enraged him.

After the war he went back to his hometown,

where he kept on working in construction. It was tough work, and though he never again was knocked out by a falling pylon, there were a lot of inconveniently timed layoffs as the fortunes of the economy ebbed and flowed over the years. Given the choice between construction accidents on the one hand and being out of work on the other, he figured he'd just as soon take his chances with falling pylons. He fell in love, married, and started a family. He was a volunteer firefighter, owned his own home, and did a fair amount of fly fishing. He had, as he used to put it, "a pretty good time, taken all in all."

The good times seem very long ago now. Mr. Wolter, for many years a widower, has been suffering from a multi-infarct dementia (caused by a series of little strokes) for over ten years, and it's been a long time since he's been able to interact with his family at all. His three children still live nearby, and if you asked them, they'd say they were a pretty close family.

Mr. Wolter's children managed to keep him out of the nursing home for quite a long while. Their mom's mother spent some time in a home just before her death, and though they were only kids at the time, they remembered the smell of stale urine and the tight-lipped nurses, and it left them with a bad attitude toward such places. That was why all three of them tried to take turns with their father's care. When Mr. Wolter was no longer able to live on his own, his house was sold and he moved in with his eldest son Paul and Paul's wife Rebecca. He lived with them for almost two years and then moved on to live with Amy, his favorite child, for better than five years. Then he lived briefly with Randy. Everybody helped as best they could. During the long and taxing time he lived with Amy, Paul or Randy would sometimes come over and spend a few days with him while she took a little break. This pattern continued for the two months he lived with Randy.

Mr. Wolter's doctors had advised against shuffling him around too often, stressing that he would do best in a stable, highly structured environment, and that changes in residence—or even changes in who was taking special responsibility for his care—could quicken the disorienting, disabling impact of his illness. So Mr. Wolter stayed about as long as possible at every stop, living with each child until the wear and tear got to be too much. Whether because of being shuffled around, or simply because of his dementia, things were particularly difficult during his years with Amy. He kept wandering away from home, and then toward the end of his stay, he became increasingly unpleasant and violent. That's when Randy agreed to take him. But it didn't work out. Shortly after he arrived at Randy's house, Mr. Wolter knocked him over, hitting him so hard that Randy broke a table as he fell. At that point, there was no help for it.

Randy took him to the emergency room for a psychiatric evaluation, after which he was pronounced a danger to himself and others and admitted to a psychiatric hospital.

After thirty days, although Mr. Wolter was still violent, the hospital staff told Randy they were going to release him. Appalled, Randy called his family doctor, who informed him that it was illegal in that state to discharge a psychiatric patient without a discharge plan—a plan for the patient's continued care. So Randy called the hospital's executive director, explained the situation, and requested a plan. The hospital then discharged Mr. Wolter to one of the few nursing homes in the area willing to take combative patients. Cedarcrest wasn't an ideal home by any means, but it was all there was. That was three years ago.

Mr. Wolter is by now extremely ill. It's been a long time since anyone has heard him say anything that could count as a clearly recognizable word, let alone put a sentence together. He can stand, but not move very much. He's been having increasing problems with swallowing his food, and he drools a good deal. It's been more than two years since he had any control of his bladder or bowels. Because his children don't think much of Cedarcrest, they've haunted the place in an effort to make sure their dad's care is okay. Randy and Paul have been spending time with him several days a week. Amy is there at least every other day. They are sad to see him so ill.

The demanding but relatively smooth routine into which matters had fallen was abruptly shattered one morning when a staff member called Amy. Mr. Wolter had developed a serious urinary tract infection and was comatose. He had been taken by ambulance to a nearby hospital—the one where Amy was born—and was on a respirator in the intensive care unit (ICU), with every effort being made to get his infection under control. Amy phoned her brothers from the hospital, breaking the bad news and assuring them that the ICU team was doing everything they could to keep their dad going. Paul and Randy, however, seemed less than enthusiastic about this course of action. Both brothers thought that what Dad would have liked best was simply to die at home. Amy, caught off guard by her brothers' attitude, opposed them bitterly. She said they were just tired of going to see Dad and wanted him to die, not for his own sake, but for theirs. She set the receiver in its cradle with a little more force than was strictly necessary and marched off to the ICU.

There, a few weeks later, he still remains. He's no longer connected to a respirator, but he has several other tubes sticking out of him. Amy is standing at his bedside, holding his hand, weeping quietly. Behind her, Paul and Randy are talking in low tones with the attending physician. Mr.

Wolter has stopped eating, and the question now is whether a feeding tube should be surgically inserted in his abdomen. The doctor has already explained that, along with more and more of his colleagues, he's reluctant to place a tube when the patient is severely demented, because it's somewhat uncomfortable and prolongs the process of dying. Amy knows her brothers wouldn't be in favor of the surgery even if the doctor recommended it and that, without it, their father won't live much longer. Amy knows too that pretty soon they'll ask her what she thinks. Standing there next to her unresponsive father, she doesn't know what she should say.

We discuss two themes in this chapter. The first is familiar: what is the role of the family in maintaining the selfhood of the demented person? Although this is a question we've never been far away from in this book, it seems particularly difficult to answer now that this final stage has been reached. This deep into the course of dementing disease, families will feel they have little to work with. It isn't merely speech and mobility that have gone; people as ill as Mr. Wolter don't seem to be themselves anymore. In fact, they don't seem to have an identity at all. Even now, however, the family has important maintenance work to do. And this work of maintaining the demented person's selfhood is crucially connected to our second theme: making decisions about health care at the end of life.

MAINTAINING SELFHOOD FOR THE DEEPLY DEMENTED

Families are a source of selfhood, consisting of perhaps the most fundamental set of relationships in the context of which people's identities are formed. Many of our core values, our strategies for coping with the world, and our basic personality styles come from our family upbringing. Many of us also find in our families the ongoing connections that reinforce and renew these parts of our identities—and even provide us with a certain degree of safety as we challenge and experiment with who we want to be.

Families start this work of forming our identities when we are babies. When we are grown, through the many subtle and not-so-subtle ways in which our intimates respond to us, they show us who they think we are: the constant mirroring we get from those with whom we interact most closely is an important mechanism by which we maintain our sense of ourselves. Families can also be a special home for human selves at the far end of life— the place where the person continues to exist even after his own body has ceased to be a home to him, even after he is no longer aware of the world around him, of those who love him, and of himself at the center of it all.

By telling stories in this book we have tried to show how people's lives can be seen as complicated, interconnecting lines of plot and character, arranged in patterns we can make sense of, and that others can understand. Understanding a loved one's life story allows us to make decisions about his health care in accordance with what the loved one would have wanted, *because* he would have wanted it; this process is an important way of keeping the patient connected to his own story. Even when the actual decision cannot or should not be solely the patient's—other people count too, after all—families can make decisions that take the ill person's character seriously. By maintaining a vivid sense of their relative's personhood in the process of making decisions that affect them all, the family can keep their relative "alive" as a member of their own intimate community, even after this person has passed beyond all knowledge of their love.

One source of the family's authority to make medical decisions for a loved one is that they have a stake in what's decided. But there is another source of decision making authority: the family's ability to reveal who their loved one has been and still is when his own actions are no longer self-revealing.

E. M. Forster's novel *Howards End* concerns what happens when the dying Mrs. Wilcox bequeaths her beloved home, Howards End, to Margaret Schlegel, an acquaintance to whom she has become very attached. The Wilcox family, appalled at the thought of an outsider taking possession of the family property, suppresses Mrs. Wilcox's will. In due course, Margaret ends up owning Howards End anyway, because she becomes the second Mrs. Wilcox. But that doesn't mean that everything has come out as it should. The wrong has not been righted, because the first Mrs. Wilcox didn't simply want Margaret to *have* Howards End—she wanted to *give* it to her as her gift, as an expression of her affection. Had the family honored her will, they would, in a sense, have acted in a way that showed something important about Mrs. Wilcox.

Not every family, of course, is equally well equipped to act in a way that expresses something significant about their loved one's personality. Families consist of individuals with separate, as well as shared, histories and hopes. While the connections among family members may be strong, they also might, as we have seen, contain very different agendas, deeply rooted suspicions, old grievances. And even when such considerations do not figure prominently in the equation, family members will grieve and love in their own different ways. What are sometimes called "moral emotions"—guilt for one, compassion for another— will be much in evidence as family members gather at the bedside. If individual needs and feelings aren't recognized and addressed, the final stages of the loved one's dying may be harmful to everyone involved.

Further, family members are not only in relationships with one another and with their demented and dying loved one—they are also in a relationship with the health care system. The tie between families and the institution of medicine is of profound importance, for it involves, at the moment of death, the family's understanding of the meaning of this event and the place of medicine in it. If all has gone well, the family will have discussed death with the patient long ago. They will have had family conferences and perhaps will have the patient's advance directive to guide them. But they must also revisit those questions in the light of their intervening experience.

Is it a legitimate goal of medicine to extend Mr. Wolter's life as long as possible? If his children really loved him, wouldn't they insist on the medical team's doing everything they could for him? What is the connection between withholding medical treatment and abandonment? What are the natural limits of human life, and how far ought we or dare we to press them? As we reflect on these general questions, we'll discuss some ideas that families can use to build their own particular paths through this difficult terrain.

FAMILY DECISION MAKING AT THE END OF LIFE

Mr. Wolter's children face decisions that are even tougher than people might think. For one thing, *everybody* in the family is on to something important in their thinking. Paul and Randy find it very hard to imagine what kind of good anyone could get out of a life like the one their dad has. He is, to put it bluntly, incapable of doing, thinking, or even feeling almost anything. Besides, his death can't be long delayed. Even if there is some value attached to living the way he is, Mr. Wolter won't be losing much if this episode of illness rather than some later one takes him away. And when you consider just what surviving this episode might cost him in terms of the pain and discomfort that accompany even minor surgery—pain he can't make sense of and doesn't understand—the meager good that such a life might be to him is surely outweighed by the rigors of being scanned, prodded, probed, injected, cut, and otherwise disturbed in order to prolong it.

These are all weighty considerations. At the same time, Amy is quite right to feel that neither brother's motivation here is completely unselfish. Dad has been difficult to take care of, and it isn't easy to regard this as rewarding work when he's so completely unable to acknowledge what they're doing. It isn't clear to either brother that the care they've been giving has really benefited him in any meaningful sense over the past few years. To one extent or another, they both feel their father has already died. "He passed away years ago," Paul says sorrowfully, "and left a disgusting stranger in his place."

If their care is costing them so much and offering him so little, what could be wrong in deciding that it's time to let Mr. Wolter go? Amy means very well, her brothers allow, but they see her as having invested so much in her father's care that she's not clear about the boundaries here. Randy put it this way: "Amy thinks that if we don't keep Dad alive as long as we can, we're telling her she's a failure, and that all her hard work went for nothing."

Randy isn't altogether wrong. Amy does feel as though she's given up too much to let her father die without a struggle. Besides, she's deeply angry at fate for doing this to Dad and to her life, and she resents her brothers a little for those five years when they stuck her with the most difficult and prolonged period of Mr. Wolter's home care. Randy and Paul, of course, are both aware of her feelings.

But they're missing some important issues that Amy sees clearly. Mr. Wolter did have an unusually deep aversion to the thought of dying—the death of his buddy in combat seemed to have been significant in forming his attitude toward such matters. While many people would see nothing to be gained for Mr. Wolter by even such a minor intervention as a feeding tube, Amy isn't at all sure *he* would see it that way. He certainly never said anything when he could still talk that made her think he'd eventually want to call it quits. In her opinion, her brothers have lost sight of who their father was. They're being guided by their own values concerning what makes a life meaningful instead of by his, and they're protecting their own interests at their dad's expense.

There are, obviously, real issues here between Amy and her brothers, and the moment before death is hardly the time to start sorting them out. People are upset, a little distrustful of each other, and under time pressure. And there's no way to play it safe. Whichever way they go, they run the risk of wronging and harming their father.

SORTING IT OUT

What should they have done? Well, they *should* have thrashed the matter out long before now. They ought to have realized that the time was bound to come when Mr. Wolter was ripe for a large-scale medical emergency. But it isn't uncommon, or unnatural, for people to put off thinking about a parent's death until they absolutely have to. It's difficult to face up to the possibility of a crisis, and very easy to put off talking about it.

Now, however, time has run out. They have to make some decisions and make them right away. What will that involve?

First, they will have to decide what kinds of concerns it is legitimate to bring to the table. The overt debate between Amy and her brothers has to do with what their father would have wanted in a situation of this kind. Everybody agrees that this is relevant to deciding what to do. But what about the hidden debate—the suspicions they have about one another's feelings? Each side thinks the others are driving their own agenda instead of concentrating on the real question, What is best for Dad? What would he have wanted for himself if only he could think and talk?

We have already pointed out that the needs and values of any one individual, no matter how ill or helpless, should not be allowed to determine how the family lives. Paul's and Randy's concerns about themselves aren't irrelevant to the decision, even if their interests do run counter to their father's. When caregivers pay heavily in time, emotional upheaval, forgone job opportunities, strained relationships, or money, this can't and shouldn't be ignored—not even if the cost to their dad is some months of his life. Mr. Wolter does have a very poor quality of life; he will die soon no matter what they try to do; medical interventions will very likely cause him some discomfort and even flat-out pain; the devotion, time, and energy that's going into his care is forcing his children to skimp—yet again—on other important family functions and personal projects. In loving families such sacrifices can be made happily and willingly during a crisis, but this is no crisis. It's a chronic, slow hemorrhage of resources that has been going on for a decade.

On the other hand, Amy's considerations can't be lightly dismissed, either. In her concern to do what her father would have wished, she isn't merely trying to second-guess what he would have said ten years ago, or what he'd say now. She's not trying to read the mind of a man whose mind is gone. Instead, she's trying to maintain her father's identity by acting for him in ways that say who he is. Now that he is past almost all forms of self-expression, she is trying to keep faith with him by expressing his selfhood for him, not only to her brothers and to the staff in the ICU, but to herself.

Her brothers are right. Much of her passion does flow from "her own issues." That fact, however, does not disqualify her feelings from consideration. Amy has put a tremendous amount of her life into her father's care, and she has done so lovingly. Losing him to death now, when there's still something that can be done to save him, suggests that the life she has struggled so hard and so long to preserve wasn't worth the effort. She rebels at that notion. She knows it *was* worth the effort,

and believes that Dad would agree with her if he
could.

So, our first decision is that all these concerns
belong on the table. What then? How can Mr.
Wolter's children have a useful, respectful conversation about end-of-life decision making for him,
when the considerations driving them are so different? When they aren't simply trying to decide
what would be best for him, but are also trying to
figure out what would be best for *themselves*, individually and as a family?

Amy, Randy, and Paul have had practice with
this kind of problem. After all, ten years ago they
did work out their "shuffling around" arrangement as an attempt to take into account their love
for Dad, their own need to have lives not completely taken up by his care, and their respect for
his strong aversion to nursing homes. That arrangement, while by no means perfect, proved
workable for quite a while. No one burned out
completely, and Dad stayed out of a nursing home
for seven years. And then, when they all had to
bow to the inevitable, they also worked out a routine at Cedarcrest for keeping him as comfortable
and happy as possible. Still, the burden wasn't divided equally and Amy is aware of that fact.

Things are even more difficult now. Ten years
ago, everyone agreed on the goal: to give Dad as
good and independent a life as he could have and
by all means to keep him out of nursing homes.

Three years ago, the goal was still to give him as good a life as he could have. What's the goal for now? Are they supposed to keep him alive as long as humanly possible, independent of costs to him or anyone else? Are they supposed to do their best to see that his care goes as he would want it? If the only alternatives are to die now or to lie deeply demented in a nursing home with a tube in his stomach, does it even make sense to talk about what he would want? Isn't it pretty clear he wouldn't want either one?

If you asked Amy to state the goal for now, she'd say it's that everybody continue to affirm clearly and powerfully that their father's life matters. You can't do that, she would say, if you let him die from conditions that medicine might be able to ease. Continuing to care for him is a way of showing the importance of his life overall. People are precious, she reminds her brothers, even when they're a major bother to other people.

Of course he's going to die sometime. We're all going to die sometime, and most men in their mid-eighties who have serious health problems will probably die sometime soon. That in itself is no good reason, argues Amy, to deny him the medical treatment that might postpone death for a while, particularly if the treatment can be provided without causing him great pain or discomfort.

And what about Paul and Randy? Paul doesn't disagree with the goal of saying clearly, in deed as well as word, that Dad's life is just as important as it ever was, even though he is demented. He agrees that their decisions now will say a lot about how much they value their father, and even about how they value the way they have been spending their lives during the past ten years.

However, Paul does want to figure out what Dad's view of further treatment would have been, now that the question is whether to be or not to be. It's all very well to say he wouldn't have jumped at either alternative, but he might have hated one less than the other. Paul thinks he knows which one his dad might have hated less. He wasn't the kind of guy who wanted life at any price so long as he could keep breathing. He took a lot of interest in improving himself and in making a better life for his family. He personally liked an outdoor life—especially if he could go fishing. It's true that he never said anything about refusing life-sustaining treatment. True too that as a volunteer firefighter he had plenty of opportunity to see the impact of high-tech medicine on badly injured people, and he could have said what he thought if he'd had any objections to it. But from his silence it doesn't follow that he thought bare biological life the most important thing in the universe or that it must always take precedence over any other consideration. He never said anything like *that* either.

Paul thinks it's reasonable to see their father's

values as complex, rich, and possibly conflicting. What he would do if he were miraculously restored to health for an hour would probably be to ask his kids what *they* thought was best for him— and for them too. If you ask Paul, Dad's track record in life gives them ample reason to think that the interests of his children were important to him, and that he would take seriously both what his family were facing and what they had already done for him.

Randy has a somewhat different take. He agrees with Amy that if Dad could be helped by something that wouldn't cause him much pain or scare him too much, they'd have to consent to it or they wouldn't be able to live with themselves. He also agrees with her when she says it's too difficult to guess what Dad would want now if only he could still want anything. But Randy thinks the operation to put in the feeding tube will hurt; and that down the road, thumping his chest and shocking him if his heart should stop will hurt; and that most of the other medical interventions that might become necessary will hurt. Maybe none of these things would frighten Dad; maybe he's too far gone for that. But he's also too far gone to be able to tell himself that the pain has a good purpose, or that it won't last long. Randy thinks it's hard to say whether his father can still be terrified, but he knows that the old man becomes agitated when Randy has to move his stiff arm to get his T-shirt on, that he's feeling something unpleasant. He thinks they could spare him more serious pain by letting him go now.

Finally, their discussions helped them come up with some goals they can all live with. They agreed on Amy's goal of acting only in ways that would honor their dad's life. They also agreed that this goal was consistent with not burdening him any more than they could help. They decided they didn't have an obligation to authorize burdensome treatment, and on further reflection they concluded *that* pretty much ruled out any kind of emergency resuscitation. They figured that since there had been no obligation to treat his infection aggressively in the first place, they were ethically safe in refusing the feeding tube now. They agreed not to authorize cardiopulmonary resuscitation (CPR) when Dad's heart stopped, as it surely would in the next few days if he weren't fed.

SECOND THOUGHTS

As the evening went by and the implications of the agreement sank in, Amy started to have some misgivings. Although in his present condition Dad couldn't understand and might be distressed by the care he would need, she never related to her father solely in terms of his present condition. In caring for a badly demented man who now recognized neither her nor himself, she considered herself a character in an ongoing story in which they both had a part.

When she was a newborn, recognizing neither her family nor herself, incontinent, unable to speak, he had changed her diaper and fed her with an eye not only to who she was, but to who she would become. Something of the same thing was happening now, only backward. Just as the future had shaped the relationship Mr. Wolter had with her when she was an infant, so did the past permeate the relationship she had with him now. She wondered if her father—when she thought of him across the full span of his life—would want that life to end just because he couldn't understand what the pain was all about.

Amy's husband, Lewis, had been working the swing shift the night the Wolter children had this discussion. It was late when he got home, but it was soon clear to him that he wouldn't be going to bed for quite a while. Amy was very upset about the way the decision had gone. She was now much less comfortable with what had seemed so reasonable to her earlier in the evening. She was also concerned that if she said anything, her brothers were going to think she had reneged on their agreement.

"Honey, are you sure Gramps would see things the way you do, and not the way Paul and Randy do?" Lewis asked.

"I'm not sure at all. That's the worst part, I

think. What they say seems reasonable, and I can see Dad buying it. But I can also see him feeling about it the way I do. What scares me the most is that my own ideas keep moving around, and I haven't got a clue as to whether that's because I'm starting to see things more clearly, or because I'm just becoming more selfish."

"Hey, you're not becoming more selfish. Nobody who knows you at all could think that—particularly not Gramps. You know what I think? I think Gramps's ideas would keep moving around just like yours do if he were trying to make this decision."

"Maybe . . . but that doesn't make it any easier. I keep flip-flopping, he'd flip-flop too, maybe even Paul and Randy flip-flop a little. The problem is how to stop flopping."

Lewis thought this over for a few seconds. "How did your dad solve problems like this before he got sick? I don't mean about medical care—I know he didn't talk too much about that. But about other important things."

"Well, I remember when he was thinking about giving up firefighting, he and I had a long talk. It was real important to him, but he had gotten the feeling that he was getting too old for the heroic stuff, that he couldn't make the same kind of contribution he used to. We had another long talk when he was first thinking about retiring from his job."

"You were his sounding board, eh?"

"No," she answered slowly. "Not really a sounding board. I was more active than that. Dad tended to be a little . . . I don't know, maybe you'd say indecisive about big decisions like those. I tried to help him know his own mind, but I guess what I really ended up doing was giving him advice. He took it, too, both times."

"You know what I think, Amy? You were helping him to know his own mind at the same time that you were making it up for him. Tell me, were those easy decisions for you?"

Amy smiled and shook her head. "They were godawful. I knew how much those jobs meant to Dad, and I also knew how strongly he felt about having to do a good job at whatever he did. But he was looking to me to help him, so he could stop flip-flopping and make a decision."

"And he trusted you to make a good one, didn't he?"

"I guess so."

"Well, I think he's trusting you now, too. I know this might sound odd, but I think you're making up his mind for him this time, just as much as you ever did. What you decide *is* his decision. That's the way he always did it."

Amy thought about it. "Yeah," she answered slowly. "That's weird but true. I never thought about it that way before. I'll tell you what, though.

I'm still just as far from knowing what to do as I ever was."

"Maybe, but now you know whatever you do decide, that's his decision, too. There isn't much danger that you won't be taking him seriously enough. No more danger than there would be if you had to make a hard decision for yourself."

The immediate effect of Lewis's idea was to help Amy get to sleep. The longer term impact was that she called her brothers the next day and asked if they could get together just one more time to go over the feeding-tube decision.

At that meeting, Amy told her brothers that she had had second thoughts. She still believed it would do more harm than good to pull out all the stops the next time Dad had a medical emergency. But she didn't think that meant they should reject every other kind of life-prolonging care for him. Instead, they should think through each treatment as it came up. In weighing its burdens against its benefits, they should take into account their best sense of what their father might have wanted, of who he was, as well as what his life was like now, and what the implications of such decisions would be for them.

"The big question about the feeding tube, I think, is what is Dad's life going to be like if he gets this procedure done? Is there anything left for him that he might still enjoy? I think there might be. Think how much he used to like to sit in the sun when he was fishing, even if the fish weren't biting. Lots of times he didn't even bait the hook. He just shut his eyes and got blissful—fell asleep half the time. He took real pleasure in that. And you all know how much he likes it when you rub his back with that little wooden back-massager. If he's agitated it calms him right down.

"I think there could still be sensations like that left for Dad. Maybe the feeding tube could give him another few months of feeling the warmth of the sun on his face and a few more nice back rubs. That's not much, I admit, but so far as we know, being dead is even less interesting."

Paul smiled a little at that, as Amy had intended he should. "He'd have to go back to Cedarcrest, you know," he said.

"I know, and I don't like that. But he doesn't know he's in the ICU now and he won't know he's at Cedarcrest. What he will know about is the sun and the back rubs, and we'll all visit him a lot, won't we? We've been so good about this for the past ten years—it can't last much longer. Let's give him this last little bit. Please."

Paul, Randy, and Amy ended up agreeing to authorize the placement of the tube, and at the same time to work out with Mr. Wolter's treatment team a good understanding of the kind of care he'd receive both in the hospital and at Cedarcrest. It was important to all of them that their father not be subjected to any further emergency care—no more ambulances, no more respirators, no CPR—but that his comfort should be a high priority and his life extended as long as it could be without having to do anything that would distress him too much.

And that's largely what happened. The tube was placed, he went back to Cedarcrest, and about two months after that, Mr. Wolter died in his sleep. In the interim, his children and their families had a good chance to say good-bye. Whereas there had been something very indefinite about Gramps's illness before, they all realized now that this was the very last chapter of his life, and they were all happy to have been in on it. Mr. Wolter got a number of very good back rubs. And it was unusually sunny that autumn.

6

Building Bridges

JEANNE QUINN is looking at her pale, red-eyed reflection in the mirror of the ladies' room at Rooney's funeral parlor. It is late in the afternoon, the second day of her husband's wake. She has been playing the grieving but composed widow to perfection—trying hard to make everybody as comfortable as possible in what they must all think of as a "difficult" social situation. Her face is startlingly white above her black dress, and for a moment, she fumbles in her purse for her makeup. But no, she thinks, she'd probably just make matters worse, and anyway, who cares? Not she, certainly, and with this realization, some fortification in her crumbles. She starts to tremble slightly, and knows that if she has to go back into the room where her husband's body is being shown and make polite small talk to a collection of people she never, ever wants to see again, she'll start scream-ing at them.

It's better in the smoking lounge, which is bless-edly empty. For the first time all day, Jeanne isn't being hovered over by family, friends, or funeral directors. She feels hollowed out, but she's stopped shaking now and is surprised by how clearheaded she is. She's reached some place where she's nei-ther acutely sorrowing nor simply numb, and cer-tain things start to strike her more plainly than they have before.

When she moved out of her last house to her present apartment, Jeanne somehow got stuck car-rying a box of books up two flights of stairs. The relief in her arms and back when she could put the box down was inexpressible, but her limbs were like rubber for an hour afterward and then ached for days. Charles's death feels something like that. She's put down a huge burden of responsibility, but carrying it at all took an enormous toll. And she knows she still has to go through the long pro-cess of taking stock of her life with her husband—particularly the last seven years, since the time when Charles started becoming a little confused.

But not now—this is no time to start raking all that up. To distract herself, she starts to think about the wake. It's been very well attended. In fact, it's positively full of familiar faces, although many of them are less familiar than they used to be. Jeanne starts to turn over all these people in her mind. Her kids have come up from Kentucky to be there, and some of her grandchildren also made the trip; her annoying sister, his annoying sister, various other friends and relations, old co-workers, people from the old neighborhood. Many of them have practically been strangers since Charles became—you know.

Everyone was on their best funeral behavior that day, though—supportive, loving, full of funny or poignant stories about Charles and what a terrific guy he had been, and all brimming over with admiration for what Jeanne had gone through in caring for him over those last seven years. Initially, surprised by the turnout, Jeanne had felt buoyed up by all the attention. But that quickly turned to a sense of depression, followed by anger. Somehow, the family's big display of support at the wake only showed how thoroughly her husband had been forgotten by his own people when things became difficult. She too has been largely forgotten. She had cast her lot with her husband, and those who shunned him shunned her too.

Almost everybody did show up for the wake, though, and some had even started to reappear during the last few weeks of Charles's life, when rumors started circulating on the family network that he didn't have much time left. Jeanne had gotten phone calls and even a couple of visits from people who had been notable only by their absence for as long as five years.

Jeanne's mouth started quivering again. What was *she* supposed to do? She got to her feet, crushed an empty Dixie cup she had been fidgeting with, and rammed it firmly into an ashtray. Where had these people been when she and Charles needed them? What were they doing here now?

There was an urn of hot water in the lounge. Jeanne made herself the day's eleventh cup of tea and returned to the rocker. For some reason the lounge was still empty. All those folks out in the other room were her family, her friends, people who had shared and created a whole life with her. She was over seventy herself, and it wasn't likely that she could trade these people in for a new set at her age. She'd been almost too busy these last few years to know how lonely she was, but now that the big distraction was gone, there was a large and jagged hole in the middle of her life. How could she reach out to her family and friends when they had all acted so disgracefully? Can I possibly build bridges to these people and still keep some shreds of self-respect, she wondered.

Thinking about her own sense of injury brought with it lots of disagreeable feelings—not all of which had to do with her relatives. The nagging sensation, long repressed, that her own care for her husband hadn't been beyond reproach, made its way into her head, and she didn't have the strength to beat it back.

Charles had been reluctant to get any medical

opinion about his growing confusion—which was typical, she thought—and Jeanne had had to push pretty hard to get him to make the rounds of doctors. She couldn't even count the times she told him, "Charles, if you've got Alzheimer's, you've got Alzheimer's. If you don't, you don't. We're both probably worrying ourselves to death for nothing. And if there is something to worry about—well, the diagnosis won't make us any worse off."

But it did. Worry gave way to waves of depression and anger that hit them both at different times and in different ways. The dementia label put a decisive end to the sexual side of their relationship. Jeanne simply couldn't summon up any interest after that, although Charles had been disgustingly interested for quite a long time. Jeanne winced as she remembered some of the bedroom scenes they had had, and how hurt Charles had been when she took over the spare room for her own.

As time went on, the fights about sex stopped, but Charles became much more difficult in other ways—prone to be loud and angry as often as not. But on thinking it over now, she felt uneasy about how willing she'd been to employ hefty doses of drugs to quiet him when he had been obstreperous, even if the drugs did tend to make him dull or half-asleep.

She had also resigned herself back then to the

fact that she'd have to put him in a nursing home at some point. She did her homework, found places that had special Alzheimer's programs, and got him on waiting lists as soon as she could. She managed to find a place for him at the first sign that he was having trouble with his bladder. Charles's sister, Annoying Susan, had objected, saying she thought it was too soon and that Charles would be disoriented, lonely, and frightened. Well, since Susan wasn't paying the piper, she didn't get to call the tune. She and Charles didn't see much of Susan after that.

It was true he seemed homesick and upset at first, although it didn't take him all that long to adjust to his new surroundings at St. Anne's. In fact, he perked up a bit for six months or so, as if he was benefiting from the Dementia Special Care Unit's program. Overall, the three years he spent there seemed to go about as well as they could—which is to say, moderately awful as opposed to unbearable. Surely, he was never neglected in any way or abused. And, she insisted to herself, she had been very much involved with his care from the start.

Actually, it would be more realistic to say that she had been very much involved *at* the start. The staff had gently hinted after the first month that perhaps she was *too* engaged in his care—"It's very understandable, Mrs. Quinn, but there's no need to feel guilty"—and that Charles wasn't being given the best chance to adjust to his new home. That was a hint she took with very little resentment. Maybe, she thought, I took it too easily. Perhaps *all* her disengagement had been too easy. Maybe Charles had gone to the nursing home too early. She could, she knew, have held out longer with him at home if she had really put her mind to it. And maybe, once he was in the home, she had cut back too quickly on her involvement in his day-to-day life.

Not that she didn't visit him religiously every week, if not more often. And it wasn't that she didn't participate in his care when she was there. She read storybooks to him and sang with him, at least while he showed any interest in these activities. After a while, though, it did seem as if she was going because of some kind of vague, social expectation that decent wives visit husbands they've placed in nursing homes, and not because either Charles or she got anything much from the visit. Even when Charles could still go on walks with her, it wasn't really taking a walk together. When she helped him eat, it didn't really seem as if it was Charles she was helping. There came a point when she went to St. Anne's mainly to see the nice people who staffed the nursing home, not to visit her husband. And as the months turned into years, she did get looser about that weekly visit; in fact, she had skipped one of her regular visits on what turned out to be the day he died.

She could almost taste the guilt, but what seemed even more bitter was her awareness that Susan had made one of her own infrequent visits that very day and, therefore, knew Jeanne hadn't been there. Jeanne's attitude toward the rest of the family had hardened pretty early on. She felt it was up to them, not her, to make friendly overtures. She had been the good and dutiful one; they had all been lax. But now she couldn't help thinking she had gotten pretty lax herself. Somehow that didn't make it any easier to deal with her relatives.

What kind of person was she, anyway, that she could be so angry at others for doing what she herself had been tempted to do? No—what she herself had done. Just who had she become over the past decade? Jeanne never used to have such feelings about people. She had thrown herself more thoroughly into her husband's care than anyone else, scorning her relatives and patting herself on the back for doing it, and at the same time she'd been perfectly willing to ignore him—really, it amounted to abandoning him—whenever she had the chance. Talk about hypocrisy! And whatever was she going to do now?

The director of the Dementia Special Care Unit at St. Anne's, Tony Eliot, walked into the lounge and sat down beside her. He hadn't seen Jeanne since the day Charles died. Jeanne had always thought of Tony as a very competent, even creative, sort of person, and anyway, he had kind eyes. He had something else, too—it was his accent, she thought. So many Americans fall for an English accent. Despite Tony's charms, Jeanne had always been a little reserved when she happened to see him at the nursing home, but somehow being here at Rooney's made it easier for her to talk freely. It wasn't too long before she was able to tell him something about her feeling that her family had betrayed her, and that she had betrayed both her husband and herself.

Tony smiled gently and nodded as if he understood. "Why don't you come to our support group meeting at St. Anne's next Saturday?"

Jeanne made herself smaller in her rocker. "I don't think so, Tony, thanks all the same. I never went once the whole time Charles was there. I couldn't see the point of it. What I needed was to *stop* thinking about what was happening—not extra chances to rehash it all. Now that he's dead, what do I want to go back to St. Anne's for? How's *that* going to help me get on with my life?"

"Well," he replied, "I think it could, you know. It's quite possible that seeing how other people have dealt with their problems—their families, their sick relatives, their own guilt feelings—could help you to cope with yours. Besides, I don't see how you'll leave off thinking about things between now and next week."

So the next Saturday afternoon, Jeanne found herself back at St. Anne's, somewhat to her own amazement. She entered the conference room quietly, a few minutes early, and found a seat at one of a group of four rather rickety folding tables that had been pushed together to accommodate the family members. The other people taking their places seemed to know one another pretty well, but Tony started the meeting by asking everyone to take a turn introducing themselves, and to say a little something about what was on their minds. Jeanne's own participation in this ritual was as brief as she could make it, and the rest of the identity parade was lost on her—she'd never been much good at names, and wasn't getting noticeably better at it as she aged. Besides, she was nervous and skeptical. How could coming to this meeting possibly help?

Jeanne wasn't so distracted, however, that she took no note of what the other people were saying. One rather dramatic-looking woman wearing a lot of silver and turquoise jewelry was talking about how hesitant she had been to take her father to St. Anne's. "Dad was always a very observant Jew. Well, I ask you—Joshua Cantor. You can't get much more Jewish. When it looked as though the only decent place that would take him was Catholic, I was worried. I thought he might think he had died and gone to heaven, only to find out that *they* had been right all along."

Jeanne laughed with the rest of them, albeit a little tremulously. She wiped her eyes and started to pick up the threads of a story being told by a tall black man named Bill.

"Flora was only fifty-four when we got the diagnosis. I'll never forget what happened right after. She didn't say a word in the doctor's office, not a word in the car on the way home. When we got back, she plain ignored all of us—ignored everything, really—for about two weeks. Spent most of her time sitting by herself in a dark room. She fixed herself something to eat most days, or we would have had to make her eat, but that was the only thing she did. She wouldn't talk to us, she wouldn't take any notice of us—she just sat.

"But then she pulled herself out of it. She came out of that room smiling and she looked good— her eyes were livelier and she was holding herself straight again. She said she was starving, so we followed her to the kitchen and watched her fix a big plate of beans and rice. She said she had 'solved' her problem. Here's what she said—she was going to commit suicide."

Nobody moved. Then Tony asked, "How did that make you feel?"

"I was shocked. We were all just appalled. This wasn't any solution. It was just a tragedy piled on top of a tragedy. We all knew she was real depressed, and then we thought that maybe she wasn't thinking straight anymore because of what the disease was doing to her. You know, that she wasn't responsible for her ideas anymore, or else she wouldn't have come up with such a thought.

"But Flora insisted she was anything but depressed. Knowing she didn't have to go through dementia had set her free. She wasn't in the dark anymore—said she felt as though she might actually be able to get some real enjoyment out of life before ending it clean."

"Well, obviously she didn't kill herself," said Tony. "In fact, I stopped by her room this morning and she's doing fine."

"Yes," Bill said, "but in a way, that's what's so awful. For me especially. I couldn't do anything to get her to give up the idea of suicide. To tell you the truth, I ran out of arguments pretty quick. How could I prove to her that what she wanted to do was wrong?

"I did tell her how much it would hurt me and the kids if she died in that way, so violently, before she really had to. But that only went so far with her. She cared about what her death would do to her family, but the way she looked at it, her fate was sealed anyway. I remember she said, 'I've got a very bad, very slow, very terminal disease. It's going to kill me unless I get in there first.'

"She had thought it all through—said that the price to the family if she had to keep on going would also be very high. She felt sure we would all come to realize just why she was doing what she had to do, and we would forgive her."

Marjorie Gibbard, sitting to Bill's left, put her hand on his and said, "I can't blame her for a second, but how awful for you."

"I thought I faced the choice of trying to get her committed or standing by while she took her own life. I couldn't stand either one, so instead I offered Flora a deal. I told her she really didn't want to die now. She was still very healthy, still with it; there was a lot of life left for her. I reminded her that we could do some of the things we had been putting off for a long time, spend more time with the children and the new grandbaby. Then, when things got bad enough that she wasn't having any more fun out of life, if she still wanted to, she could kill herself."

Jeanne was riveted by this story. She had totally forgotten her own worries, and was completely caught up in Bill's. "Is that what happened? She decided to put it off?"

"Not exactly. The idea tempted her, but she was worried that she wouldn't be able to tell when would be the best time to kill herself. If she waited too long, she might get too confused to do it right and she'd maybe end up in a coma or something. She wanted to set some definite date, maybe six months in the future, have a specially good half-year with the family, and then take a lot of sleeping pills.

"So that's how things stood for about five months. Then I played my last card. I reminded her that she was still doing as well as she had been when all this started, and anybody could see it wasn't time yet. I told her that if she'd promise me not to take her own life, I'd do it for her. I gave her my word. So long as she seemed to be having a decent ride, we'd all help her have it to the fullest. When the time came that she needed to go into a nursing home or if she stopped being herself—if she became violent all the time, or abusive, or promiscuous—well, I promised her I wouldn't let her go through that.

"At first, she didn't believe a word I said, though she was touched, you could tell. She wasn't sure I had the guts, and anyway, she didn't think she could ask me to take the risk. But I swore up and down I'd do it. I told her I'd seen how the guarantee that she could escape this thing was giving her strength and peace, and that I didn't want to take that away from her. I said that if loving her as much as I could meant killing her, well, I would love her as much as I could. I said I'd have her with me longer if she trusted me to do it instead of doing it herself." Flora's husband fell silent.

"I'd have said all that to my wife," a burly man in a blue workshirt said abruptly. Marjorie Gibbard looked uneasy.

"Well, it's not so bad now. She doesn't seem too unhappy, really, though she went through some bad patches. I think she likes the things you do here in the special unit, Tony. But I know that if she knew back then what her life would be like now, she'd've been furious that I talked her out of suicide. I couldn't have killed her. I knew that when I promised I would. I knew I had to save her life. But what kind of life did I save for her? I feel as guilty as sin about the whole thing."

The turquoise-jewelry woman, Anne Cantor, jumped on this. "But whose life are we talking about here, anyway? I mean, the Flora who used to hate the idea of being demented is gone now. She's not the Flora who's living here at St. Anne's. The old Flora, the first one I mean, really is dead—at least that's how it seems to me. She just didn't die by taking sleeping pills."

"I've heard that idea before, but hard as I try, I honestly can't see it that way. If I did, what would bring me back here all the time to visit with her? I come because she's my wife and I love her, even though I let her down."

"Right, Bill's right," Barbara Johnson broke in. "When I finally brought my father to St. Anne's, he thought one of the other residents here was my mother. I guess she was flattered or lonely or something—or maybe she thought *he* was *her* husband, I don't know. Anyway, they wanted to move into the same room together, and her family thought that was okay! They said what did it matter now, as long as it made them happier. But it *wasn't* okay. My father adored my mother. He was faithful to her his whole life—faithful to her memory after she died! If I had let him move in with this woman, it would've been like saying I didn't care about who he had been. But it was my job to care. That's just what I'd been doing ever since he became ill—trying to keep alive his connections to who he had been his whole life."

Everybody started talking at once, but the babble died down and Tony seized the chance to say, "Go on, Barbara."

"Well, he made a fuss, but now he doesn't seem to mind. He's not doing very well overall, though. Maybe it would have been better for him, kept him happier, but I just couldn't see it. When we bring people we love here, are we just supposed to forget about who they used to be?"

At the foot of the table a man who'd said his name was Dwayne Bailey looked up from his coffee. He ran his hand vigorously through his hair and asked, "How is being with this woman any different from marrying again?"

"I don't think Dad ever would have married again. I've told you how much he loved my mother. But that's not really the point. It *wasn't* as though he were marrying again. He thought it was my mother. He would have been terribly upset if he had known."

"Would have, maybe, but never could in the real world. Isn't that the point?"

"No, it's not the point at all. I don't believe this stuff about him not being the same person anymore. It's up to me to help him be himself, the person he's always been, because he can't do it on his own now."

Marjorie Gibbard spoke up again. "I don't think it's a matter of who your dad is, but of what's best for him now. Last year there was a badly demented woman here and a rather less confused man who—well, they paired off. Luz and Emmett—remember?" Some of them did. "He asked permission for them to live in the same room, but both their families insisted the staff keep them apart. Emmett actually pined away. Every time I saw him he was sadder and frailer. He died very soon after." There were nods and murmurs. "He died of a broken heart."

Barbara was quiet for a moment. "I still think I did the right thing. I know I have to look out for what my father needs now, and it doesn't bother me very much to play along with some of his delusions. But this one would be right down at his core. If who my father was his whole life means anything, it means that he doesn't treat another woman as if she were my mother."

She blinked the tears out of her eyes. "But I still feel just like Bill does. Guilty as sin. Sometimes I catch myself just wishing he would die, because I don't seem to be able to do anything to keep him in touch with who he was. And *that* makes me feel guilty too."

Jeanne felt brave enough to speak up. "Don't

think it stops after they die," she said. "I never felt so bad about everything as I have since Charles died."

"You mean, there's no relief to look forward to."

"Not so far. I did what I told myself was my very best for Charles, but now I see I was just fooling myself the whole time. And I was mad at everybody else in the family because nobody but me would do their best for him. Mostly, they just dropped us like we were a pair of hot bricks."

The man in the blue shirt, Roy Pyne, frowned at that. "Wait a minute, Jeanne—is that your name, Jeanne? Why did you think you had to do your *very* best for Charles? I mean, why wasn't it enough just to do a good job caring for him?"

"I did do a good job."

"But you feel lousy about it. Why do you feel lousy about doing a good job when we're talking about something incredibly hard to do—something that tears us up emotionally and goes on for years? And you got no help from the family. I think you're hard on yourself. Why isn't doing a good job enough?"

"It certainly doesn't feel like enough. I feel like I let him down, and I don't know how I'm ever going to be able to forgive myself." Jeanne worked to keep her mouth steady.

"Did he make you promise never to put him in a nursing home—stuff like that?"

"No. He was more the 'I don't want to be a burden on my family' type."

"Well, there you are. I mean, if Barbara's right and we're supposed to be faithful to the person we used to know and all, then you ought to be feeling just great about yourself. It seems like you not only did a good job, you did the only kind of job he would have wanted you to do."

"There's another thing that occurs to me about your problem." Amy Wolter spoke quietly. "Your family and friends. Have you thought about what your husband would have felt about them? I mean, would he have felt resentful?"

"No, it took a lot to get him to resent anything. He'd probably have thought they had done about all they could. He certainly wouldn't have wanted me to be mad at everybody. And neither do I, really."

There was a knock on the door, followed by trays of cookies, courtesy of the kitchen. People took advantage of the break. When they had come back to the table, Tony said, "Well, as happens most times we're together, we're hearing a fair amount about people feeling guilty because they aren't sure they've done enough, or done what's right. Who's had any success in trying to deal with their feelings of guilt?"

Dwayne replied first. "It's funny how that works sometimes. I thought I had done a good job being realistic, both about my mother and about myself. I didn't feel guilty, exactly, about the decisions I'd made for Mom, or about how involved I've been in her care. But something was really bothering me, and it came out when I visited her here. I'd be short with her, and I found it very easy to be upset with the staff. Even with you, Tony, as I recall."

"Well, once or twice." Tony smiled.

"I did feel guilty about that. I knew I wasn't behaving very well. But here's the odd part. One evening, I was getting ready to go to sleep, just trying to relax and let my mind go blank, when I had the strangest experience. It was as if I could hear someone speaking to me, saying, 'Let her go.' Just that. 'Let her go.' "

"Weird," said Amy.

"You bet. But I knew right away what the voice was telling me. It wasn't about how my mother was becoming demented and I had to stop pretending she wasn't; I had accepted that. What was getting to me—what I hadn't accepted—was the *way* she was becoming demented. I don't know what I'd been thinking, but I guess I had an image in my head of something like 'dignified dementia,' some picture of the way my mother would do it— the same way she always did everything, with a kind of style. Once I let go of that, I didn't have to be so angry and upset with her anymore. I could just let my mother be who she was. It's helped a lot."

Roy said, "That reminds me of the time I saw the women at the day care center singing 'You Are My Sunshine.' I think I've mentioned that in this group before. Somehow, where—and who—they were didn't seem so terrifying all of a sudden. They were just people with a bad illness that people sometimes get. That helped a lot when I was taking care of my wife. It also helped with my own fears about myself, to tell the truth."

"I've got a story, too," Marjorie Gibbard said, "but it's one I've only been able to tell lately, since Alan's mom has been here at St. Anne's. Since then I've been able to get some distance on the period when she was staying with us—on what it did to our family life as well as the effect it had on each of us personally.

"The thought that seemed to help me the most during the time she was actually living with us had to do with staying connected to myself. I sometimes see myself from the outside, as if I were a dear friend I cared about very deeply. Thinking about myself that way when I'm in trouble helps me to remember that I really like myself, that I'm interested in where I'm going and what I'm doing with my life.

"I've been doing this—I don't know, this connecting—thing for years. But lately it's turned into something different. It sort of expands the connection idea, I guess. Anyway, I was taking a shower one day, right after Alan's mom had moved here, and I was feeling beat and miserable, both because I felt we'd finally failed her in a big way, and because I knew we weren't anywhere near the end of it. I was trying to tap into my 'connection' feeling, when it hit me that there was more than myself here to be connected to. It seemed to me that everything I had been going through, the whole saga of Alan's mom's illness and what it had meant to the family, was immensely *interesting*. Sad, painful, awful, guilt-making, yes—but mainly interesting.

"What the family had been going through together was really fascinating, in a way: figuring out how to help a person we all loved to write the last chapter of her life. Now, maybe it sounds a little cold-blooded to call it interesting—as if I were taking all that pain and putting it under a microscope, but that's not what it's like. It's like the reason the old 'connection' strategy works for me is because I'm absolutely fascinated by what I'm connected *to*. I know I couldn't have felt this way when I was in the middle of the worst of it. But I sort of wish I could have. And I'm glad I'm feeling this way now. It really helps."

"How does it help?" Jeanne asked.

"Well, I guess I should say it helps me. I haven't been able to get Alan to see what I mean, or maybe it just doesn't work for him. My kids understand it better. Anyhow, when I can see my life as bound up in things that really matter, that are enormously—well, interesting—it makes everything easier. It makes me feel as if the pain and guilt I'm suffering are a part of something momentous—not just meaningless, useless misery. My energy is being expended on something fascinating. And I can't tell you how much easier it's been to forgive myself and other people for mistakes and weaknesses since I saw how interesting we all are."

Some people around the table that day—Roy Pyne and Amy Wolter, in particular—found Marjorie's story intriguing; others seemed puzzled by it and pressed Marjorie to explain the full history of the idea, starting with the baby she'd given up for adoption. Even for those who were too caught up in guilt and grief to take the perspective Marjorie was offering, it helped a little to think they might not always feel the way they felt now, and sometime in the future they might be able to look back on this time and say that it was interesting. The group talked on for another hour or so, with old problems being discussed and new stories told, and then everyone went back to their lives, and to their continuing struggle with dementia.

But Jeanne went home with something she hadn't had before. She returned to her third-floor walk-up tired and hungry, but with her head full of what had happened that afternoon at St. Anne's. The story that poor man told about his wife! How absolutely awful. And something Amy had said about Charles not being the kind of person who'd resent the family for dropping out of sight these last few years. She did want to reconnect with her family, but she felt so hurt by them. Maybe if she thought of it as a way of doing what Charles would have wanted, her own pride would be salvaged and she wouldn't feel quite so bad.

Water just about set to boil now, Jeanne noticed. Sauce ready for the microwave. Isn't there some fresher lettuce in here? And what did the woman at St. Anne's mean when she talked about being connected to yourself and interested in what was happening around you? Jeanne didn't know quite what to make of that, but she didn't think she'd forget about it anytime soon. What had happened to her over the past decade *was,* she decided, deeply interesting, and she was very interested in what was going to happen next. She was struck by the positive feelings that came from giving herself permission to think of her life in this way.

Angel hair pasta is ready so fast, that's what's nicest about it, she thought, as she sat down to eat. She poured herself a glass of red wine, lit a candle, and continued to think over the day. Jeanne had been thoroughly uninterested in support groups while Charles was alive. She had always felt she needed whatever space she could get between herself and Charles's illness, and that going to a group to hear other people talk about dementia for hours didn't seem like a very smart way of getting a break. Besides, she didn't think that they'd be dealing with the problems that bothered her the most. Now that Charles was dead, though, and she had seen what went on in the group, she was beginning to change her mind. It did her good to see these people trying hard to stay true to themselves, like when Barbara kept her father from moving in with that woman. That was being true to her own self and true to her father's self, too. And Dwayne, when he told himself to let go of his expectations for how his mother should "do" dementia. What was that, if not a creative way of accepting what couldn't be changed? All of them had been trying to see things clearly, and to help each other do that too. She liked how they gently pushed each other to think about what they were going through. That was what Roy had done for her after she told them how guilty she felt. It wasn't that Jeanne agreed with everything the other people in the group did or said. But she was impressed and comforted by what they were trying to do. She thought she'd go back. Maybe, after she washed up her dishes, she'd give Susan a call.

In this book, we've attempted to offer you who are dealing with the same kind of problems as Jeanne something of the help she's starting to find in the group at St. Anne's. The stories here are not your stories, and the ways in which our characters have thought and acted are not necessarily your ways of thinking through and acting on the challenges before you. Yet the stories do show people in situations that might seem familiar to you, and we hope that by reading them you begin to feel less on your own. We hope they leave you better equipped to understand and respond to the problems of caring for a relative suffering from a dementing disease. Such caring can play havoc with your finances, your home, your career, your health, and your feelings. It can also put enormous pressure on what you may value the most—your sense of integrity and goodness. None of these disturbances can be eliminated. But by joining your own reflections and hard work with those of others—among your family, among friends, or even in the pages of a book—some of them can be made less difficult. With luck and grace, it may be possible to come through this time intact—even, perhaps, a little kinder and wiser.

Appendix

Getting Practical Help: Some Places to Start

OUR STORIES have tried to highlight the many ways in which Alzheimer's challenges our values, and to provide some examples of how people have tried to cope with those challenges. Caregivers may find that their understanding of the nature and importance of safety, or truth-telling, or dignity, or promise-keeping, or of life itself comes under fire as they face dementia in company with their relatives; these have been our chief concerns in this book.

But we don't at all mean to suggest that these are the only kinds of problems family caregivers will face. As we've shown in these stories, caregivers will also need to know how to get hold of good medical services, particularly for diagnostic purposes; Alzheimer's often evades detection for too long. Too, caregivers will need to know who is there to help them as they try to meet the responsibilities of the rest of their lives; where can people turn to find reliable sources of respite? They will often be faced with the need to help a person of fading competence put their financial and legal affairs in order: which lawyers specialize in work of this sort, and how may they be found? In many instances, caregivers will need to consider various forms of assisted living or nursing home placement for their relatives: how may this be done most responsibly and most efficiently? And caregivers will also, quite often, need each other: where are the peer groups that can support caregivers emotionally, be a source of further caregiving stories and tips, and represent the interests of people with dementia and their families to the wider society? In this brief Appendix, we have pulled together addresses, phone numbers, and sites on the internet that caregivers may find useful as they try to meet these needs.

WHAT'S AVAILABLE BY TELEPHONE?

There may be more help than you think, and a good place to start to find out is via the telephone. *Eldercare Locator* is a referral service run by the National Association of Area Agencies on Aging. Callers are asked the name, address, and zip code of the older person, and are then told how to contact Alzheimer's service agencies and other relevant groups in their locality—e.g., their own Area

Agency on Aging or State Unit on Aging. Callers are also directed to the **Alzheimer's Association.** Eldercare Locator can be reached at 1-800-677-1116 on Monday through Friday, from 7 A.M. through 11 P.M. The Alzheimer's Association itself is in Chicago; call either (312) 335-8700 or 1-800-272-3900. There is a special number for the hearing impaired as well: (312) 335-8882. Address for mail: 919 North Michigan Avenue, Suite 1000, Chicago, IL 60611-1676. Another Chicago area–based national organization is the **Alzheimer's Disease and Related Disorder Association.** Their phone number is (874) 933-1000; their address, 4709 Golf Road, Suite 1015, Skokie, IL 60076. The ADRDA coordinates a network of self-support groups with chapters throughout the country; a call to the national office will let you know how to contact the group nearest you.

There is also a phone number for the office of the **National Association of State Units on Aging**—(202) 898-2578—but you can check your own phone listings under "State Government Agencies." The state unit will refer you to your **Area Agency on Aging,** if there is one close to you. Your state unit or area agency may well be a very useful source of referral to many readily accessible resources—support groups, health organizations that specialize in dementia diagnosis, and adult day care services that specialize in Alzheimer's. You might also find it useful to call the **National**

Association of Adult Day Care Services at (202) 479-6974.

The *Alzheimer Society of Canada* is located in Toronto, and can be reached at (416) 925-3552, or, within Canada only, at 1-800-616-8816.

OTHER NUMBERS AND ADDRESSES

- BENJAMIN B. GREENFIELD NATIONAL ALZHEIMER'S LIBRARY AND REFERRAL CENTER, 919 North Michigan Avenue, Suite 1000, Chicago, IL 60611-1676, (312) 335-5767. The Alzheimer's Association numbers—(312) 335-8700 or 1-800-272-3900—can also be used to gain access to the library.

- ALZHEIMER'S DISEASE EDUCATION AND REFERRAL CENTER (ADEAR), National Institute on Aging, P.O. Box 8250, Silver Spring, MD 20907-8250, 1-800-438-4380, Fax (301) 495-3334.

- THE JOSEPH AND KATHLEEN BRYAN ALZHEIMER'S DISEASE RESEARCH CENTER (ADRC), Box 2900, Duke University Medical Center, Durham, NC 27710, (919) 684-6274.

- NATIONAL INSTITUTE ON AGING INFORMATION CENTER, P.O. Box 8057, Gaithersburg, MD 20898-8057, 1-800-222-2225.

If you have access to the Internet, there is a great deal of information available. For example, the ***Alzheimer's Discussion Group*** provides a forum for caregivers, researchers, and other interested folks to discuss issues related to Alzheimer's. Sponsored by Washington University's ***Alzheimer's Disease Research Center,*** the discussion group is offered in both a regular and a digest format. The regular format allows you to participate in discussions, while the digest format may be better if you don't care to be "interactive." To subscribe, e-mail to:

majordomo@wubios.wustl.edu

Messages (other than subscription requests) should be sent to

alzheimer@wubios.wustl.edu

You can also check out their home page at:

http://www.biostat.wustl.edu/alzheimer

The Public Policy Division of the National Alzheimer's Association runs a list which transmits their "Public Policy Alerts" via e-mail. To subscribe, send a message with a subject line reading "E-mail Advocate" and a body stating your e-mail address to:

Jennifer.Zeitzer@alz.org

DIAGNOSTIC RESOURCES

Because getting a diagnosis can often be so difficult, statewide networks of regional diagnostic and assessment centers have been developed in California, Florida, Illinois, Maryland, New Jersey, Ohio, and Pennsylvania; other states may be involved in developing diagnostic networks of their own. We got this list from the very useful *Alzheimer's Day Care: A Basic Guide,* by David A. Lindeman, Nancy H. Corby, Rachel Downing, and Beverly Sanborn. It was published by the Hemisphere Publishing Corporation in 1991. *Alzheimer's Day Care* is particularly rich in addresses for state agencies around the United States supporting Alzheimer's day care and related respite programs with state funds. However, phone numbers and addresses can change relatively quickly; we noticed many alterations as we prepared this appendix.

California, as befits its status as the most populous state, has several Alzheimer's Disease Diagnostic and Treatment Centers:

- UNIVERSITY OF CALIFORNIA AT DAVIS–NORTHERN CALIFORNIA ALZHEIMER'S DISEASE CENTER
  Alta Bates Medical Center
  2001 Dwight Way
  Berkeley, CA 94704
  (510) 204-4530

- UNIVERSITY OF CALIFORNIA, DAVIS, ALZHEIMER'S
  CENTER
  1771 Stockton Boulevard
  Suite 2005
  Sacramento, CA 95816
  (916) 734-5496

- UNIVERSITY OF SOUTHERN CALIFORNIA/ST. BARNABAS
  ALZHEIMER'S DISEASE DIAGNOSIS AND TREATMENT
  CENTER
  675 South Carondelet Street
  Los Angeles, CA 90057
  (213) 388-4444

- SOUTHERN CALIFORNIA ALZHEIMER'S DISEASE
  DIAGNOSTIC AND TREATMENT CENTER
  Rancho Los Amigos Medical Center
  University of Southern California
  12838 Erickson Street, Building 301
  Downey, CA 90242
  (310) 401-8130

- UNIVERSITY OF CALIFORNIA, SAN DIEGO,
  ALZHEIMER'S RESEARCH CENTER
  9500 Gilman Drive
  La Jolla, CA 92093-0948
  (619) 622-5800

- PROGRAM FOR ALZHEIMER'S DISEASE CARE AND
  EDUCATION (PACE), UNIVERSITY OF CALIFORNIA,
  SAN FRANCISCO
  1350 Seventh Avenue, CSBS-228
  San Francisco, CA 94143-0848
  (415) 476-7605

- STANFORD ALZHEIMER'S DIAGNOSTIC AND RESOURCE
  CENTER
  c/o Palo Alto VAMC
  Psychiatry 116A3
  3801 Miranda Avenue
  Palo Alto, CA 94304
  (415) 493-5000

- UNIVERSITY OF CALIFORNIA, SAN FRANCISCO/FRESNO
  ALZHEIMER'S DISEASE CENTER
  1343 North Wishon Avenue
  Fresno, CA 93728
  (209) 233-3363

- UNIVERSITY OF CALIFORNIA, IRVINE, ALZHEIMER'S
  DISEASE DIAGNOSTIC AND TREATMENT CENTER
  Medical Plaza, Room 1100
  University of California, Irvine
  Irvine, CA 92717-4285
  (714) 824-2382

Florida offers clinics at the following locations:

- MEMORY DISORDERS CLINIC
  12901 Bruce B. Downs Boulevard
  Tampa, FL 33612
  (813) 974-3100

- UNIVERSITY OF MIAMI MEMORY DISORDERS CLINIC
  University of Miami School of Medicine
  1400 N.W. Tenth Avenue, Suite 702
  Miami, FL 33136
  (305) 243-4082

- ALZHEIMER'S AND MEMORY DISORDERS CLINIC
  4300 Alton Road
  Miami Beach, FL 33140
  (305) 674-2543

- DIAGNOSTIC PHYSICIAN'S 1 CLINIC
  P.O. Box 100383
  Gainesville, FL 32610
  (352) 395-0111

Two **Illinois** diagnostic centers:

- ALZHEIMER'S DISEASE AND RELATED DISORDERS
  CENTER
  Southern Illinois University School of Medicine
  P.O. Box 19230
  Springfield, IL 62794-14113
  1-800-342-5748 (within Illinois)
  (217) 782-8249

- RUSH ALZHEIMER'S DISEASE CENTER
  710 South Paulina Street
  Suite 8 North
  Chicago, IL 60612
  (312) 942-4463

Institutes in **New Jersey** include:

- ALZHEIMER'S EVALUATION PROGRAM
  Center for Aging
  42 East Laurel Road
  Suite 3200
  Stratford, NJ 08084-6843
  (609) 566-6843

In **New York,** the diagnostic and treatment centers are called Alzheimer's Disease Assistance Centers (ADACs), and are sprinkled throughout the state:

- ADAC OF LONG ISLAND
  99 South Street
  Suite 106
  Patchogue, NY 11772
  (516) 935-1033

- ADAC OF CENTRAL NEW YORK
  550 Harrison Center
  Suite 120
  Syracuse, NY 13202
  (315) 464-6097

- ADAC OF THE FINGER LAKES
  274 North Goodman Street, Box K3
  Suite 401
  Village Gate
  Rochester, NY 14607
  (716) 442-7319

- ADAC OF NORTH EASTERN NEW YORK
  SUNY at Plattsburgh
  Sibley Hall-227
  101 Broad Street
  Plattsburgh, NY 12901-2681
  (518) 564-3377

- ADAC OF WESTERN NEW YORK
  Deaconess Center
  1001 Humboldt Parkway
  Buffalo, NY 14208
  (716) 886-4400

- ADAC OF BROOKLYN
  370 Lennox Road
  Brooklyn, NY 11226
  (718) 270-2452

- ADAC OF THE HUDSON VALLEY
  Burke Rehabilitation Hospital
  785 Mamaroneck Avenue
  White Plains, NY 10605
  (914) 948-0050, ext. 2375 or 2419

- ADAC OF THE CAPITAL REGION
2212 Burdette Avenue
Troy, NY 12180
(518) 272-1777

Diagnostic resources in **Maryland** vary by region. Central Maryland and the Maryland/Washington corridor have many diagnostic facilities, most located within community hospitals. In western Maryland, contact the Alzheimer's Disease and Related Disorders Program at Washington County Hospital, 322 East Antietam Street, Suite 305, Hagerstown, MD 21740, (301) 582-3080. In eastern Maryland, try the local Alzheimer's Association chapter or a community hospital in Baltimore or Wilmington.

Pennsylvania has twenty comprehensive geriatric assessment programs located throughout the state, offering full programs for memory disorder diagnosis, treatment, and caregiver support. Contact the Project Office of the Alzheimer's Disease Initiative for the Commonwealth of Pennsylvania, 400 Market Street, Rachel Carson State Office Building, Harrisburg, PA 17101-2301, (717) 783-1550.

FURTHER ETHICS RESOURCES

And finally, if you are interested in pursuing in greater depth the kind of ethical questions we've explored here, you might find it helpful to know more about the *Hastings Center,* 255 Elm Road, Briarcliff Manor, NY 10510. The Hastings Center publishes the *Hastings Center Report* six times a year; it is one of the very few publications focusing on ethics which aims to achieve both scholarly excellence and wide accessibility in its articles. Memberships in the Hastings Center, carrying a subscription to the *Report* as well as other benefits, are available for $55 a year ($42 for seniors and full-time students).

Sources and Suggestions

AS WE HAVE ALREADY ACKNOWLEDGED, our greatest help in preparing this book came from the family members who shared their stories with us and helped us to understand what they were going through. We also benefited enormously from our professional consultants. But a third source of help came from other writers' books and articles. We want to acknowledge these writers, and also offer our readers suggestions for further reading.

Three books in particular were useful in the writing of *Alzheimer's: Answers to Hard Questions for Families.* One is *The Caregiver's Guide: Helping Elderly Relatives Cope with Health & Safety Problems,* written by Caroline Rob with the help of Janet Reynolds, and published by Houghton Mifflin in 1991. The second is *Broken Connections,* a book in two parts written by Liduin Souren and Emile Franssen, and published by

Swets and Zeitlinger in 1994. The third is *The Thirty-Six Hour Day,* by Nancy L. Mace and Peter V. Rabins, published by the Johns Hopkins University Press in 1982. *The Thirty-Six Hour Day* is something of a classic in this field, and it is particularly full of interesting (if occasionally controversial) ideas: Roy Pyne in Chapter 3 got the idea for stamping Marie's checks "void" from reading this book.

Regarding the importance of families in helping people form their personalities and hold themselves together as life goes on, we have learned a good deal from Salvador Minuchin's book, *Families & Family Therapy,* published by Harvard University Press in 1974.

The work of Tom Kitwood and his co-workers from the University of Bradford in the United Kingdom has also been very important to us as we thought about the relationship between what happens inside the head of a person suffering from dementia and what happens in their day-to-day surroundings. Kitwood's opinion is that dementia arises both from damage to the brain and from a social environment that is disrespectful to elderly people. Many of his articles have been printed in a journal called *Ageing and Society.* A particularly interesting piece he wrote with Kathleen Bredin, called "Toward a Theory of Dementia Care: Personhood and Well-Being," was published in 1992 in volume 12, pages 269–87, of *Ageing and Society*.

Another article very much worth reading in the same volume of *Ageing and Society* is Steven Sabbat and Rom Harré's "The Construction and Deconstruction of Self in Alzheimer's Disease," which is on pages 443–61. If you're interested in the discussion between Anne and Bill in Chapter 6 about who Flora really is, you will find that Sabbat and Harré say some very useful things. We are also indebted to them for the story of Henry the lawyer, which you read in our Introduction.

We learned a lot about the kind of world confronting Marie, who figures importantly in Chapter 3, from reading Diana Friel McGowin's touching story of her own struggle with dementia, *Living in the Labyrinth,* which was published in 1993 by Elder Books.

We have also drawn heavily on the work of Margaret Urban Walker in preparing this book. We made particular use of two of her essays, both published in *Metaphilosophy*. One is "Moral Luck and the Virtues of Impure Agency," published in 1991 in volume 22, pages 14–27. The other is "Moral Particularity," published in 1987 in volume 18, pages 171–85.

We read Stephen Post's book, *The Moral Challenge of Alzheimer Disease,* in manuscript and found it interesting; Johns Hopkins University Press published it in 1995. Another book you might like is Beverly Coyle's novel about Alzheimer's disease, entitled *In Troubled Waters,* published by Ticknor & Fields in 1993. And a nurse-administrator and family caregiver, Barbara Bridges, has written *Therapeutic Caregiving: A Practical Guide for Caregivers of Persons with Alzheimer's and Other Dementia Causing Diseases,* published in 1995 by BJB Publishers, 16212 Bothell Way S.E., Suite F171, Mill Creek, WA 98012.

We've also used a little of our own earlier work. We first discussed the *Howards End* example from Chapter 5 in an article called "Guided by Intimates," which appeared in the *Hastings Center Report* in 1993, in volume 23, number five, on pages 14–15. We discuss other matters concerning families and caring for aging relatives in the fifth chapter of our book *The Patient in the Family,* published by Routledge in 1995.

Printed in the United States
by Baker & Taylor Publisher Services